Peter Kaš

Colour illustrati
Krzysztof Wołowski

An Ordinary Day in 1945

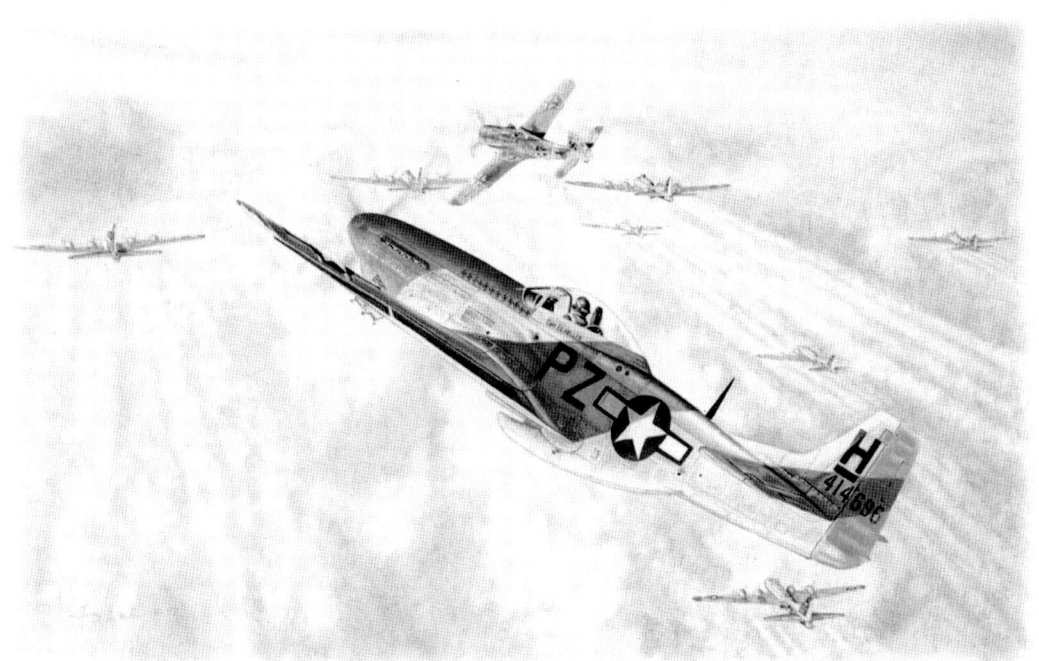

STRATUS

Published in Poland in 2005
by STRATUS
Artur Juszczak, Po. Box 123,
27-600 Sandomierz 1, Poland
e-mail: arturj@mmpbooks.biz
for
Mushroom Model Publications,
36 Ver Road, Redbourn,
AL3 7PE, UK.
e-mail: rogerw@mmpbooks.biz
© 2005 Mushroom Model
Publications.
http://www.mmpbooks.biz

All rights reserved. Apart from any fair dealing for the purpose of private study, research, criticism or review, as permitted under the Copyright, Design and Patents Act, 1988, no part of this publication may be reproduced, stored in a retrieval system, or transmitted in any form or by any means, electronic, electrical, chemical, mechanical, optical, photocopying, recording or otherwise, without prior written permission. All enquiries should be addressed to the publisher.

ISBN 83-89450-22-4

Editor in chief
Roger Wallsgrove

Editorial Team
**Bartłomiej Belcarz
Robert Pęczkowski
Artur Juszczak**

DTP
**Robert Panek
Dariusz Karnas**

Translation
Wojtek Matusiak

Colour Drawings
Krzysztof Wołowski

Printed by:
*Drukarnia Diecezjalna,
ul. Żeromskiego 4,
27-600 Sandomierz
tel. (15) 832 31 92;
fax (15) 832 77 87
www.wds.pl marketing@wds.pl*

PRINTED IN POLAND

Table of contents

Author's preface 3
Introduction 4
Morning intrigue: Luftwaffe vs. 2nd TAF. 5
Propellers and jets 14
8th AF – Mission #859 18
    Task Force I 18
    Task Force I fighter escort 22
    Task Force II 26
    Task Force II fighter escort 30
    Task Force III 42
9th AF vs. I/JG 2 45
Annex 48

Acknowledgements: (for written accounts and materials):
Christer Bergström (S), Jim Perry (USA), Richard C. Penrose – 339 FG (USA †), Jozef Chovanec (SVK), Donald Caldwell – JG 26 (USA), Eric Larger (F), Karol Steklý (SK), David E. Brown – Experten Decals (USA), Jan Zdiarský (CZ), Robert D. Elliott – 92 BG Assn. (USA), Bill Jones – 20 FG (USA), Andreas Berg, Ace Johnson – 91 BG Assn. (USA), Klaus Schiffler (G), Matthew Smith (USA), Wido Schlichting (G), Kevin M. Pearson (USA), Chelius H. Carter – 364 FG Assn. (USA), Robert H. Powell Jr. -352 FG Assn. (USA), Thomas L. Thomas – 96 BG Assn. (USA), Mario Isaac (G), Troy White (USA), Roger Feller – 385 BG Assn. (USA), Dr. Frank J. Olynyk (USA), Thomas W. Mooney – 464 BG (USA), Capt. Ret. Harry F. Howard – 339 FG (USA), 390th Memorial Museum Foundation (USA), Dirk Lehrmann (G), Don Magness – 485 BG (USA), Phillip Duffrasne (B), James R. Starnes – 339 FG (USA), Bill Varnedoe – 385 BG, Ján Malovec (SVK), Richard Goyat (F), Martin Veselý (CZ), Edward N. Gibbs – 467 BG(USA), Trevor Allen – B-26 Marauder Historical Society historian (UK), Will Louie – 354 FG (USA), Merle Olmsted – 357 FG Assn. (USA), Mike Mucha (PL), Christer Landberg (S), Jack T. Curtis – 367 FG Assn., Charles J. Tighe (USA), Bruno Peters (USA), Jaromír Kohout (ČR), Boris Súdny (SK), Buck Pattillo (USA), Allan Hillman (UK), Guy Ries – 385 BG Assn., Ken Wells (USA), Bob Baxter (UK), Ken Wells – 355 FG, Steve Coates (USA), Gary Ferrell – 34 BG Assn., Tom Thacker – 52 FG Assn., Tálosi Zoltán (HU), Steve Brew – 41 Sqn (CH), John Cripps – 198 Sqn (UK), Serge Bonge – 350 Sqn (B), Robert G. Schimanski – 357 FG (USA), Dale E. Karger – 357 FG (USA), Dr. Jakob Mayer (A), Tom Ivie (52 FG), Jiří Rajlich (CZ).

Get in the picture!

Do you have photographs of historical aircraft, airfields in action, or original and unusual stories to tell? MMP would like to hear from you! We welcome previously unpublished material that will help to make MMP books the best of their kind. We will return original photos to you and provide full credit for your images. Contact us before sending us any valuable material: *rogerw@mmpbooks.biz*

Author's preface

This work discusses aerial combats fought over Europe on 2 March 1945. It should not be considered the final and ultimate study of the events it describes. While finding out details of the encounters between the 8th AF and German fighters, the research proved so wide that it was possible to piece together the mosaic of other aerial engagements of the fighting powers.

This work mentions aircraft and fates of famous aces, as well as those of less known airmen who have carried out their duty. Ordinary men on both sides displayed uncommon courage, facing the confusion and fear of their daily duties. Therefore, I would be glad if this work could be treated as small monument to those men who fought and died unknown.

In my research I was able to contact many co-workers, yet not all units have been confirmed by historians, not all archival materials survived to date, not all documents are available in archives (that is why Soviet units are not mentioned), and most of the eyewitnesses have, sadly, already 'flown their last sortie'. Still, those whom I was able to contact, gave their testimony of the day that was quite usual for others, but so exceptional for them that they kept the memory of its details for over half a century. This is their story…

Title page:
"All The Way" painting by Troy White. Capt. Ed Heller of 352 FG in his P-51D, serial 44-14696, "HellEr Burst" (PZ-H) closes on the tail of Uffz. Guenther Schultz, FW 190D-9 W.Nr. 500569. "White 14".

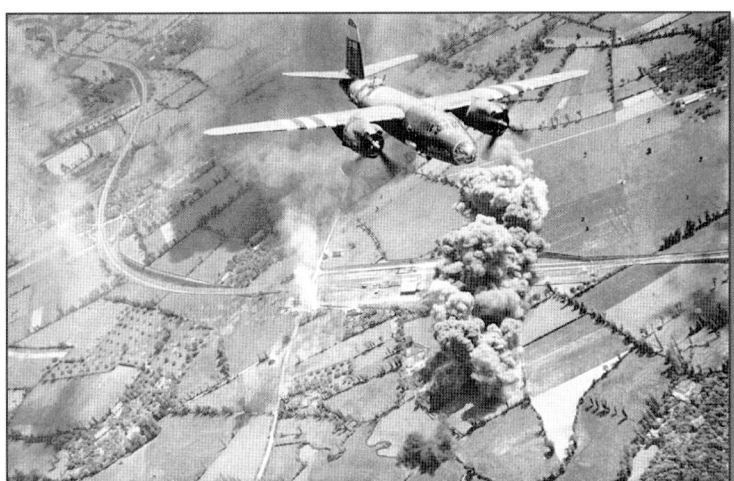

Left:
9 AF Marauder attacking targets in occupied Europe.
9 AF Assn.

Introduction

The date of 2 March 1945 does not appear particular in any way, compared to other days. A typical day of the seventh year of the war. And yet, the day was different and more interesting. The day saw one of the last 'blood-lettings' of the German Luftwaffe. One of the last major encounters of the opposing air forces.

In the west, Allied forces fought to establish control of the western bank of the Rhine. The US 3rd Army captured Trier. In the east, with

Right:
Gun camera shot from 330 FG aircraft, showing the destruction of an Me 262.
via 339 FG Assn.

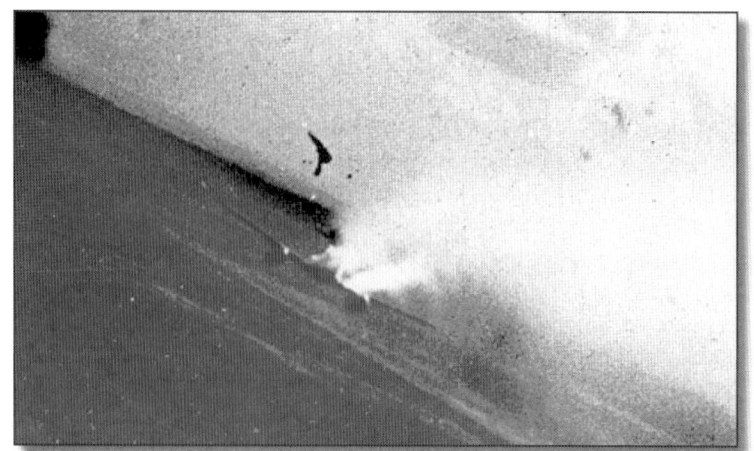

help from partisan forces, Soviet troops crossed the Slovak mountains and headed towards Bratislava and Vienna. Further north, Soviet troops reached Breslau (Wrocław).

Experienced "war horses" on the German side, and old soldiers among the Allies, already knew that the end of the war was imminent. But the supreme headquarters of the Luftwaffe did not accept the possibility of a defeat, and the German piston-engine fighter pilots were constantly experiencing the discomforting feeling under the guns of US Mustangs, Thunderbolts and Lightnings, or RAF Tempests and Spitfires, that enjoyed ten-fold superiority.

Pilots of the 'turbines'[1] did not have to worry about their tails while in the air. They could always accelerate and dictate the terms of engagement. But it was the high speed that made landing difficult. The approach and speed reduction procedures were longer, so the pilots were more prone to being hit during landing than ever before. This was one of the reasons why the Allies left nothing to chance, and the bases of the jets were visited almost daily. Also any report of 'propellerless aircraft' flying across the lines was never left without reaction. 'Rat patrols' took off immediately to knock the enemy out of the sky.

Right:
Ar 234s of III/ KG 76 lined up on their base.

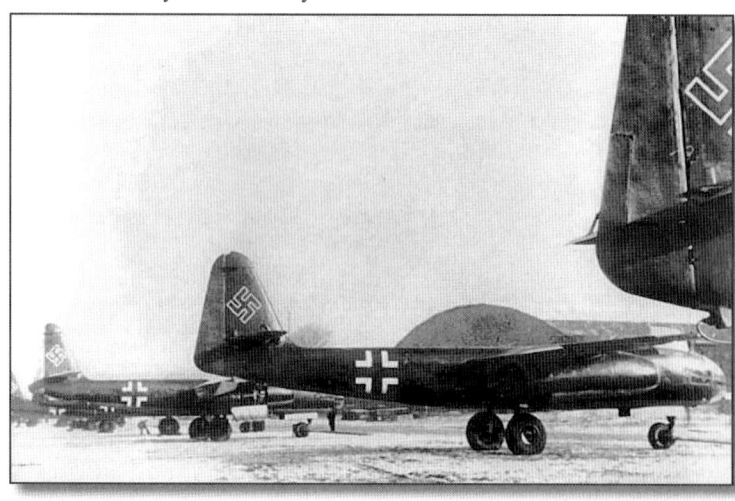

[1] Nickname of the first operational bomber with jet engines.

Morning intrigue: Luftwaffe vs. 2nd TAF

An Ordinary Day in 1945

Friday 2 March 1945. Aircraft took off from forward airfields of the 2nd Tactical Air Force, RAF, for patrols over the front line. Their task was to repel any raid by jet bombers, the activities of the latter constantly growing. And indeed that day 21 Arado Ar 234 Blitz German jet bombers left Achmer[2]. Two machines belonged to Stab Kampfgeschwader 76, led by Oblt. Robert Kowalewski, and the remaining 19 machines of III

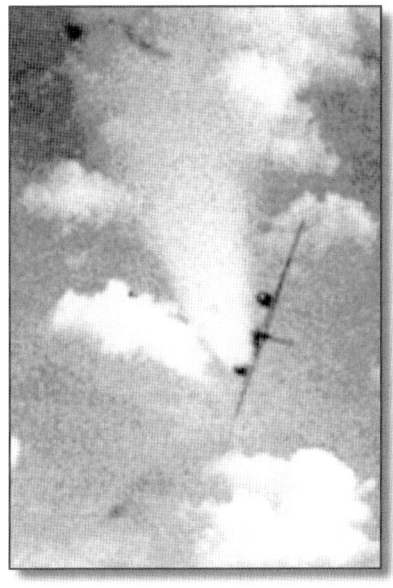
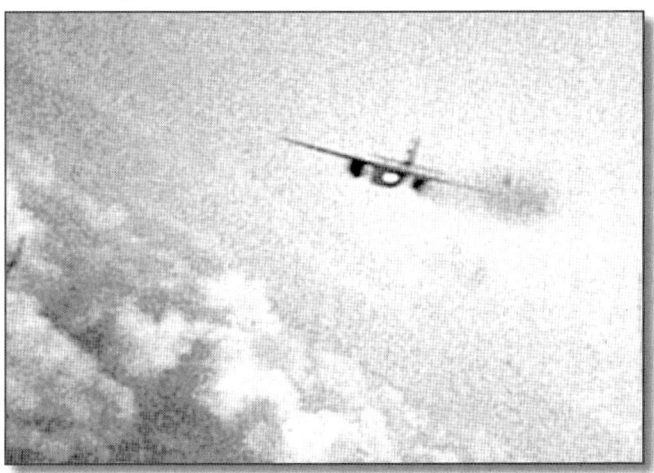

Gruppe KG 76, led by Major Franz Zauner who had replaced Gruppenkommandeur Major Hans-Georg Bätcher on 26 February 1945. Their task was to attack Allied positions in the area of Maastricht-Aachen-Jülich. The bombers were escorted by a group of aircraft from JG 27, namely 71 Messerschmitt Bf109K-4 fighter aircraft from III and IV/JG 27 from Hesepe and Achmer airfields, and older Bf109G-14s from II/JG 27 from Hopsten.

Above the target, British tanks at Düren, the Luftwaffe met RAF Spitfire XIVs of 41 Sqn and Tempests of 222 Sqn RAF. The British intended to intercept the attractive prey, the jets, but the German fighters had their tasks and wanted to fulfil these as best they could. In the ensuing air combat both sides scored victories and suffered losses. Overall, the Allies fared better.

III Gruppe KG 76 lost two machines on 2 March 1945. The Arado Ar 234Bs from 9/KG 76, flown by Oberleutnant Sutterlin and Leutnant Eberhard Rögel (F1+QT [W.Nr. 140178]), were both shot down. Lt. Rögele was killed at Hamnermühle, 3 km west of Recke, while Oblt. Sutterlin managed to bale out uninjured. A third Arado Ar 234, F1+EY (W.Nr.140166), was damaged in the combat. Its pilot, Oblt. Arthur Stark, Einsatzstaffel

Above and left: Gun camera pictures showing the destruction of an Ar 234 bomber. via 339 FG

[2] *9/KG76 moved to Münster-Handorf on 17 December 1944, and remained there until March 1945. It is not known if that Staffel still operated from this airfield on 2 March 1945, or had it joined the rest of the Gruppe at Achmer by then.*

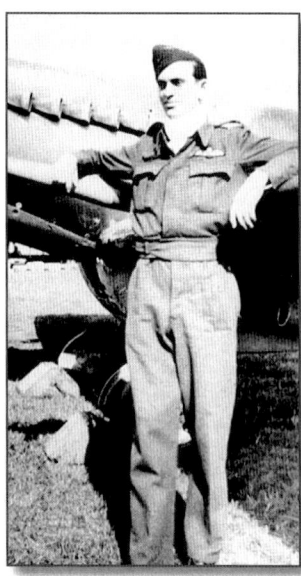

F/Lt. Dennis J. "Danny" Reid, 41 Sqn.

via. A. Hillman

veteran, managed to perform an emergency landing on the German side, at Lippstadt. The pilot walked out of his aircraft with only minor wounds.

After the combat two British pilots claimed jet bombers shot down: F/Lt Dennis J. 'Danny' Reid[3] of 41 Sqn and F/Lt George W. Varley of 222 Sqn RAF. It was F/Lt G. W. Varley, flying Hawker Tempest (EJ882, ZD-E), who downed Lt. Rögel and one 109 which he claimed as destroyed upon return to his base. He said that 'his' Arado exploded in mid-air.

Clearly, Oblt. Sutterlin was shot down by D. Reid. Damage of an Ar 234 at 07.55-08.10 was claimed by W/O T. B. Hannam of 222 Sqn. This may have linked with the machine of Oblt. Stark, but that is just a hypothesis.

The course of the entire action was described by F/O Vic Murphy of 130 (Punjab) Squadron RAF, who noted in his diary:

'I was flying from Eindhoven, Netherlands in 130 Squadron together with a Belgian Squadron which made up 125 Wing commanded by Group Captain 'Johnnie' Johnson (famous RAF war ace). When 'Johnnie' flew with the Wing I was usually his 'wingman'. On this particular day (March 2nd), I was leading a Section of Spitfires – noticed an oncoming dot ahead, approaching tremendously fast! Within seconds it passed approx 500 ft below me (our combined speed would have been 1,000 mph) I noticed German Air Force markings on a black fuselage. It was a twin engine jet!! I immediately radioed my location, the compass reading of the German plane and the height. This information was acknowledged by one of our pilots in that section. It enabled the pilot to gain good height above the German and enabled the pilot to dive on the German jet to match its superior speed and shoot the German jet (Arado 234) down...'[4]

This account links with the victory claimed by 41 Sqn's F/Lt Reid. We can find more information in Pierre Clostermann's book of memoirs, 'The Big Show'[5]

'Another poisonous day. Snow, wind. Visibility nil; flying was quite impossible. However, G.C.C. maintained two sections of Tempests at immediate readiness - one from 486 and one from 56 - together with a section of Spit XIVs from 41 Squadron. There was a time for one pair of Spits took off, followed at least three minutes later by the rest. A quarter of an hour later these last four came back and landed, not having been able to join-up in the clouds. They told us, however, that the first two had jumped a German jet-aircraft.

We got the remainder of the story that evening in the bar, when the pilots of 41 were distinctly pleased with themselves and let nobody forget it. Flying Officer Johnny (Dennis) Reid D.F.C., shortly after he had scrambled and as he was patrolling Nijmegen bridge at 10,000 feet, had spotted one of the very latest and rarest Luftwaffe planes - an Arado 234 - sneaking into our lines at ground level. Diving straight down, flat out, ignoring the risk of his wings coming off, Johnny succeeded in catching the bastard in a turn, fired at him point blank and gently landed him in flames less than 100 yards from Broadhurst's H.Q. at Eindhoven.

We naturally retorted that this particular Hun must have been very keen to commit suicide. Besides we'd seen Reid's plane after he landed: his poor Spit's wings were buckled like a concertina, all the paint had come off the

---

[3] Danny J. Reid died of cancer on 1 May 1993 in Melbourne at the age of 72. It was for the action on 2 March 1945 that he was awarded the Distinguished Flying Cross (DFC).

[4] Vic Murphy was shot down on 19 April 1945 in Spitfire XIVe RN203 during a mission over Celle.

[5] This memory is mistakenly dated 25 February 1945. On this day also one Ar234 was shot down by P-47s. It was Ar 234 (F1+MT) W.Nr.140173 crashing near Seegesdorf. But Danny Reid claimed only one Ar234 and it happened on 2 March 1945. On February 25, 1945 Reid claimed an Fw190D-9 at 08.15 over Rheine a/d.

surfaces, the rivets had sprung and the fuselage was twisted. Good for the scrap heap!'

German bombers were not left unescorted, however. The first to come to their defence were 12 Messerschmitts, probably from II/JG 27. They were followed immediately by the pilots from III and IV Gruppe. The British claimed four Bf 109s destroyed. Three machines were credited to three F/O pilots of 222 Sqn: H. E. Turney (NV674 ZD-V), Australian, McAuliffe (NV670 ZD-X) and V. W. Berg (EJ873 ZD-R). The fourth 109 was downed by F/Lt Varley mentioned above.

II/JG 27 was lucky, and it lost only Oblt. Wolfgang Herkner (born 12 June 1921) who fell to British fighters with his G-14 somewhere over Achmer, Saerbeck. Upon their return Lt. Anton Wöffen and Uffz. Hans Stenglein, both from 6/JG 27, claimed destruction of two Tempests. This apparently happened at 07.51 West of Osnabrück and at 07.59 East of Rheine. Wöffen noted this victory with only a small remark in his memories: *"During an aerial battle I got my fourth victory, it was a Tempest. I didn't feel any joy over this victory either. I couldn't help thinking that it could have happened vice versa as well."*

One of these must have been the Tempest V (EJ691) of 80 Sqn RAF, flown by Norwegian Capt. Olav Ullestad. During the encounter of 122 Wing with some 16 Bf 109s and Fw 190s, Ullestad's machine was hit at 07.50 north-west of Rheine by one of the 109s. The pilot baled out and was taken prisoner. British documents make no mention of any other lost Tempest.

While the bombers used their superior speed to evade attack, their escort suffered serious losses. As opposed to the relatively fortunate II Gruppe, its sister units had much less luck. III Gruppe of JG 27 lost three Bf 109K-4s in combat. Between Tecklenburg and Saerbeck Fw. Karl Schaffhauser (born 22 February 1919 at Rücksdorf) from 12 Staffel, Fh. Karl-Heinz Eidam (b. 18 April 1920 at Düsseldorf) from 9 Staffel, and Uffz. Erich Schulz (b. 16 February 1920 at Seedorf) from 11 Staffel of III/JG 27 were all killed. Their death was avenged by their colleagues from the same Gruppe. Oblt. Heinz-

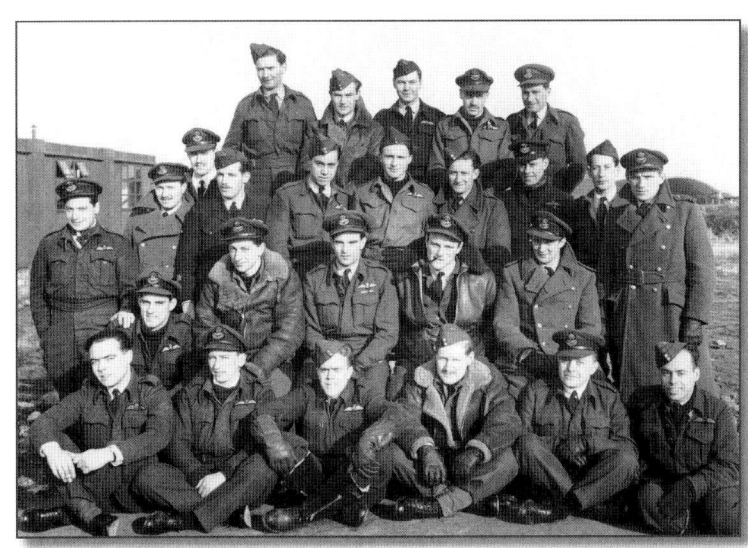

Group photo of 222 Sqn. pilots. F. Salter via A. Lamb

An Ordinary Day in 1945

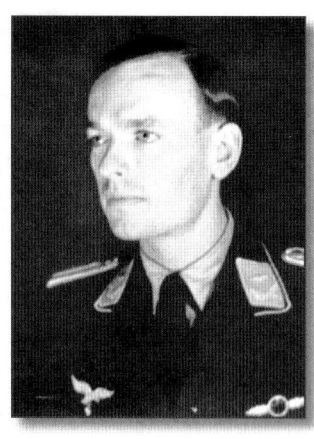

Lt. Anton Wöffen, Staka 6 JG 27.

[6] *Clifford Harper Mottershead, Flying Officer, RAFVR no. 164378, 41 Sqn, flew Spitfire XIV, RN123. He is buried at the cemetery at Maastricht, Limburg, Netherlands (row 4, grave 164).*

[7] *This Typhoon credited as shot down is either a case of a misidentified type or of an overclaiming. Two machines of 198 Sqn were attacked by two Fw 190D-9s. One was apparently shot down in flames. But this British machine is believed to have been shot down in error by a USAAF P-51. As regards the 'long-nose' D-9s, these could have been machines from JG 26 whose pilots claimed an encounter with P-47s, Spitfires and Tempests. Tempest and Typhoon looked pretty similar, and could have been confused.*

Günther Hennig from 10/JG 27, Uffz. Heinz Durchdewald from 12/JG 27 and Fw. Werner Schreck from 10 Staffel claimed at 07.43, 07.50 and 08.00, respectively, three Spitfires shot down. Two of the machines (probably the first and the third claims) were certainly from 130 Squadron RAF. They fell 10 km south-east of Rheine, while the victim of Uffz. Durchdewald crashed at Ibbenbühren. These two machines, serial nos. RM750 and RM914, were flown by F/Lt G. G. Earp and F/O N. W. Heale, respectively, who ended up as German PoWs. The third claimed Spitfire was probably serial no. RN123 of F/O C.H. Mottershead[6] from 41 Sqn. The pilot was killed, and he is buried at Maastricht.

It is worth quoting the Operations Record Book of no. 125 Wing. Under 2 March 1945 it includes the following note:

'To-day for the first time since we arrived at this resort we were able to take to the air as planned in the early morning. Both squadrons were airborne at 07.19 hours, the Wing Commander leading 130 Sqn on a sweep and were warned when in the Enschede area that Huns were in the Rheine area. This is what all the pilots had been hoping for so off they went and the Wing Commander caught a glimpse of a nice gaggle of mixed 190s and 109s about 1,000 feet below and then the fun started. The W/Cdr dived down with 130 Sqdn and quickly got on the tail of a Hun and in a very few minutes the latter had decided he had had it and out he came complete with parachute. The Wing emerged with 5 destroyed, 3 probables and 3 damaged plus 1 destroyed claimed over the R/T by F/Lt Earp. This was not achieved without loss as F/O Heale and F/Lt Earp both of 130 Sqdn did not return. F/O Heale was seen diving with a Hun on his tail and those who saw him last were not happy about his chances of having got away with it. George Earp had trouble with his engine, probably as a result of the scrap and nursed it back some way but could not make it and is presumed to have crash landed somewhere in enemy territory. Before doing so he sent his claim to the Squadron and claimed a 190 destroyed. F/Lt Samouelle believes he probably destroyed the Hun who shot down F/O Heale. He saw Heale turning inside the Hun but the former suddenly straightened up and the e/a got in a quick burst. Sammy was by that time able to get in a burst at the Hun which followed Heale's aircraft down in a vertical dive, both a/c streaming glycol and smoke. He got some strikes on another Fw190 but was not able to finish off the bird.

After this hectic beginning to the day the pilots had a relatively boring job giving some cover to Mediums on Kevelaer and Geldern. This was uneventful, the bombing was not seen owing to cloud. Later in the day 6 aircraft gave cover over base to the V.I.P. and needless to say it was uneventful.'

The fourth Gruppe of JG 27 shot down one Typhoon[7], claimed over Achmer by Lt. Manfred Stechbarth from 13 Staffel. This was his first and last victory. Immediately following this success his machine was hit and Stechbarth was wounded, but survived. Pressure from the British fighters knocked two more Bf 109K-4s out of the sky. Gefr. Alfred Pölz (born on 28 June 1925 at Steyr, 14/JG 27) was killed at Münster, while Gefr. Robert Sonnet (15/JG 27) survived, albeit wounded. Additionally, Lt. Horst Nitschke (born on 24 September 1924 at Glogau/Głogów), Staffelkapitän of 12/JG 27, was killed in his machine, when his K-4 suffered a malfunction during take-off and crashed into a parked Bf109G-10 (W.Nr. 490646). Altogether, IV/JG 27 lost four pilots that day.

Two Typhoons of no. 198 Sqn were attacked near Vynen by two Fw 190Ds (and of course Bf 109s) during their mission against ships north-west of Neuss. One of them was shot down in flames. This was Typhoon Ib MN354 (TP-K) flown by W/O W. A. Livesley[8], who was killed. According to British sources this loss was caused by an American P-51 that apparently hit the Typhoon. Subsequent opponents of IV/JG 27 included pilots of 350 Squadron, its combat described below.

Two more Typhoons were lost by the Royal Canadian Air Force (RCAF). Machines RB285 'Z' of 438 Sqn and MN144 of 439 Sqn were hit by Flak in the area north-east of Dülmen and Appelhüsen, without connection with the described encounter. The pilot of the former, F/Lt D. J. Heard, was taken prisoner, while F/Lt L. C. Shaver[9] from the latter was killed.

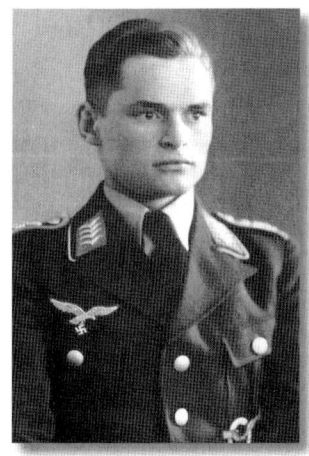

Oblt. Ernst-Heinrich Herkmer. Born on 12 June 1921 at Marburg a.d. Lahn/Kassel. Died in the air battle against British fighter on 2 March 1945 as a pilot of II./JG 27.

via Bundesarchive

According to the Operations Log of 439 (CAN) Squadron, the second mission of the day was flown by the following pilots: MN144 – F/L Shaver L.C., RB477 – W/O Roach R.J., RB198 – F/L Breck A.W., PD608 – F/O Harrison J.L., SW443 – F/O Roberts J., MN936 – F/O Bullock J.W., PD451 – F/L Jackson S.C., SW420 – W/O Horrocks L.J. Their task was to bomb ground targets. The mission took place between 10.55 and 11.40. The document gave the following description of the loss:

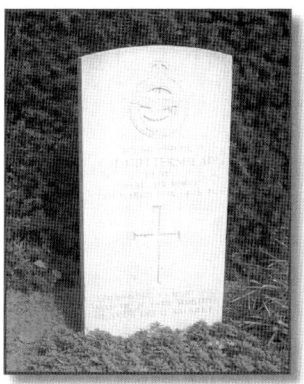

The whole Wing was airborne on the same target that 439 Squadron attacked earlier in the morning, the railway and marshalling yards at Buldern, on the Dulmen-Munster line; 500 lb. 11 second delay tail-fused bombs were carried. The aircraft took off in pairs and climbed through 8/10ths cloud over base. The Wing formed up and set course at 7000 feet, 439 Squadron acting as top cover. The trip to the target was uneventful, and the Squadron attacked in order. 439 Squadron was the last squadron to go down, using a 60 degree dive. No results were observed.

After the attack, F/L Shaver & F/L Breck attacked a loco and 15 plus cars, with a claim of 4 cars damaged; considerable light Flak was encountered and F/L Shaver was seen to be hit, flick on his back, dive into the ground and burst into flames in the area E8546. F/L Breck climbed up through 10/10ths cloud and returned to base alone, landing at 12:05 hours.'

Another Typhoon, RB281 5V-X 'Nicky' from 439 Sqn RCAF, flown by F/O Hugh Fraser, was forced to land north of Eindhoven aerodrome. The pilot flew over the aerodrome and after the forced landing he left the cockpit unscathed. The aircraft was repairable. Another Typhoon of 44 Sqn emergency landed at Eindhoven field with pilot McCarthy in the cockpit.

[8] *William Arnold Livesley, Warrant Officer (Pilot), RAF no. 1451431, buried at Venray War Cemetery, grave no. VII. C. 2.*

[9] *Clarence Lyell Shaver, Flight Lieutenant (Pilot), RCAF no. J/17058, Reichswald Forest War Cemetery (ca. 5 km south-west of Cleves) grave no. 21. H. 18. Until his death he had flown 66 operational sorties in 80:15 hours during his second combat tour, giving a total of 202 operational sorties in 171:55 hours.*

An Ordinary Day in 1945

That day III Gruppe of JG 26 'Schlageter' left its base at Plantlünn with 21 Fw 190D-9s to practice formation flying. At 08.00 the German pilots were attacked from above by a group of some seventeen Tempest, Spitfire and Thunderbolt aircraft.[10] The combat was fought at altitudes of 3,000-7,000 m. Focke Wulf Fw 190D-9 'black 10' (W.Nr.400257) of Uffz. Walter Hähnel from 10/JG 26 (born on 11 January 1924 at Meißen), crashed in the area north-west of Ibbenbüren, Pl.Qu. GQ 5-1, killing the pilot. This was the only loss of JG 26 in the encounter.

On the Allied side the engagement saw Spitfire XIV pilots from the already mentioned 130 and 350 (Belgian) Squadrons, 125 Wing. They encountered some 20 Fw 190 and Bf 109 aircraft. This shows that the combat had expanded. The 109s were those from JG 27. The Belgians were the first to enter combat, aiming at the Messerschmitts. Their attack was successful: F/Lt R. Hoonaert[11], P/O L. Lambrecht[12], F/Sgt J. Groensteen[13] and F/Sgt E. Pauwels[14] were each credited with a Messerschmitt destroyed.

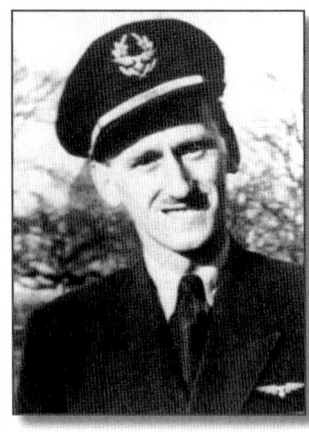

F/Sgt. E. Pauwels, 350 Sqn RAF.
S. Bonge via A. Bar

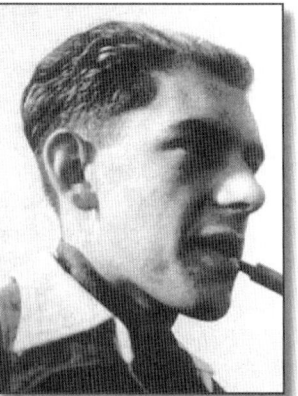

F/Stg. J. Groensteen, 350 Sqn RAF.
via s. Bonge

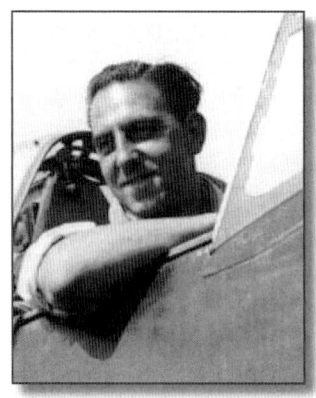

Right:
P/O L. Lambrecht, 350 Sqn RAF, Friston, May 1944.
S. Bonge via P. Deman

[10] *The information about Allied aircraft types comes from the historian D. Caldwell. However, no Thunderbolt unit active that day was identified (even if only the 9th AF can be taken into account).*

[11] *Roger Hoonaert (RAF no. 128392), this was his only victory in WWII. Born at Etterbeek (Brussels) on 4 April 1921. On 4 September 1939 he took up a voluntary 2 year service with the Aéronautique Militaire Belge and was admitted to the 82nd Promotion at the Pilot School of Wevelghem. 13 May 1940 saw his unit leaving for France. Via Marseille the Pilot School passed to the airfield at Oujda in the French Morocco. He escaped to Great Britain, where he arrived on 5 August 1940 and joined the Belgian Forces in Britain. Posted to RAF Depot at St Athan (13 August 1940), he transferred to the EFTS at Odiham (2 November 1940) where he started initial training. On 15 February 1941 he joined the SFTS at Ternhill, followed by the OTU at Grangemouth (2 June 1941). F/Sgt Hoornaert, freshly graduated, received a posting to 234 Sqn where he arrived on 17 July 1941. Further postings saw him joining no. 2 Delivery Flight (10 September 1941), 66 Sqn (6 April 1942), 60 Sqn (15 June 1942) where he was commissioned, 91 Sqn (25 January 1943). Rested, and promoted to F/O, Hoornaert joined the Aircaft and Armament Experimental Establishment at Boscombe Down as test pilot (10 September 1943). Posted to 349 Sqn (20 March 1944), he left for RAF Belgian Depot (24 March 1944), and finally joined 350 Sqn on 22 June 1944, becoming a flight commander. Shot down on 4 April 1945, he crashed near Lingen and was made PoW. Repatriated on 12 May 1945, he was posted to 106 Personnel Receiving Centre at Cosford. Next day saw him joining no. 30 Belgian Rest and Leave Centre Camp at Goring. Posted to HQ Transport Command (19 September 1945), he was discharged from the RAF on 18 April 1946. He joined Sabena airlines and eventually finished his carreer with Sobelair. During his last flight with Sobelair, he made a succesful crashlanding at Sant Cruz Airfield in Tenerife with a Boeing 707-329 (c/n 17627 OO-SJE) when the nosewheel collapsed while landing, the plane being destroyed by fire. Fortunately there were no victims. Roger Hoornaert died at L'Escala (Spain) on 28 September 1997. Awards: Knight in the Order of the Crown with Palm, Croix de Guerre 1940 with Palm, French Croix de Guerre 1940 with Bronze Palm, 1939-1943 Star (info via Guy De Win).*

Then came the time for 130 Squadron. Its pilots claimed 4-1-2 Fw 190s, including confirmed destroyed by F/Lt G. G. Earp (his subsequent fate has been described in the section discussing III/JG 27), F/Sgt P. H. T. Clay, F/Lt Ch. J. Samouelle and W/O Joseph A. Boulton. A 109 damaged was claimed by F/Lt Samouelle, while a probable and a damaged was credited to the Australian W/O J. T. Turnbull. W/C G.C. Keefer RCAF, who led the sweep, also claimed a 109.

Claims from this encounter have to include that made by S/L Robert B. Cole from 3 Sqn, who claimed an Fw 190 destroyed in the Dülmen area, while flying his Tempest V (NV775).

As mentioned above, 130 Sqn was also hit, losing two Spitfires. As yet unidentified pilots of III/JG 26 were credited with two P-47s destroyed, and one probably destroyed[15].

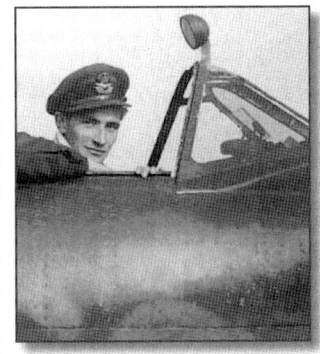

F/Lt. R. Hoonaert, 350 Sqn RAF.
S. Bonge via A. Bar

As already mentioned, one German Ar 234 bomber was damaged. Unfortunately, German records do not quote individual loss times. However, during the afternoon hours two pilots of 222 Sqn fired at an Ar234 during a sweep in the Rheine area. Damage to the bomber was claimed at 14.10 5 miles east of Lingen by F/O R.A. Carson. This might link with the damaged F1+EY (W.Nr.140166) of Oblt. Artur Stark.

That was not the end of German jet bomber activity, though. Another mission was flown by Ar 234 bombers of KG 76 between 16.20 and 17.31 in the Bürg area. This information comes from the flying log book of Lt Anesten, held at the Luftwaffe Museum in Berlin-Gatow. The German pilot flew Ar 234 W.Nr.140589.

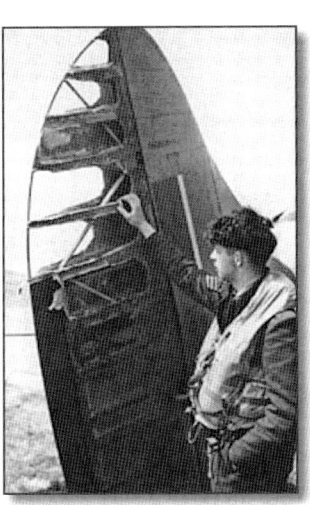

S/L Robert Bob Cole, 3 Sqn RAF.
via S. Brev

[12] Louis 'Boum' Lambrecht (RAF no. 1899871), prior to this victory on 2 March 1945 he had already scored twice. Upon his return from the sortie on 21 February 1945 he was credited with an Bf 109 destroyed and another damaged at Paderborn. Born in Rotterdam on 23 August 1917, Ludovic took up a voluntary engagement at the Pilot School for two years and was admitted to 76 Promotion (1 September 1937). On 1 September 1939 he re-engaged for one year. The country being invaded by the Germans, he passed with his unit to France (15 May 1940). On 20 August 1940 he returned to Belgium. He left Belgium for France (25 May 1942) and was arrested at Verona in Spain (14 June 1942). Imprisoned at Barcelona, Saragossa, Irun, he finaly arrived at Miranda on 29 July 1942. Released on 19 April 1943, he was sent to Gibraltar. He arrived in Britain on 24 July 1943. He joined the Belgian Forces in Britain (4 August 1943) and was posted to the AéM Depot. Training saw F/Sgt Lambrechts passing to no. 1 RAF Depot (15 November 1943), RAF College – SFTS (27 December 1943) and 57 OTU (28 March 1944). He was posted to 350 Sqn where he arrived on 30 May 1944. After a short posting to 26 Sqn (5 September 1944), he returned to 350 Sqn, serving in it until the end of the war. After the war he joined Sabena. He was killed in an aircraft crash (Sabena Boeing 707-329 00-SJB) at Berg (near Brussels Airport) on 15 February 1961. His awards included: Croix de Guerre with 2 Palms, Knight – Officer in th Order of the Crown, Kinght in the Order of Léopold, Médaille de la France Libérée (info via Guy De Win).

[13] Jacques A.H. 'Pichon' Groensteen (RAF no. 1299861), born on 23 October 1922. As a civilian escapee he reached Britain on 20 May 1940. He applied at the Belgian

An Ordinary Day in 1945

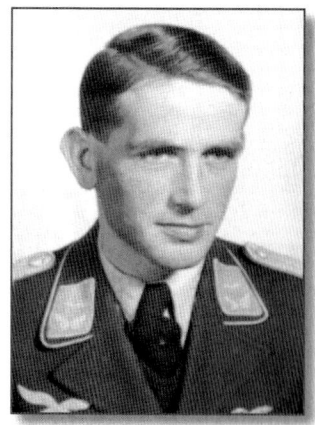

Hptm. Friedrich Wilhelm August Abel. Born on 28 November 1919 at Wintenberg/Westfallen.
via Bundesarchive

Embassy on 27 August 1940 and was posted to Tenby Camp for military training. He applied for a transfer to the air force, and was moved to the Belgian reserve until 7 August 1941. On 29 September 1941 he was posted to the Aircrew Receiving Centre and commenced his flying training (86A pilot promotion) at no. 5 ITW Torquay (3 October 1941), then at no. 6 EFTS Sywell (20 December 1941), 22 EFTS Newmarket (1 May 1942), RAF Cranwell (20 May 1942), Infirmary/A Sqn/Fl 2 Eastbourne (20 June 1942), 58 OTU Grangemouth (29 September 1942), following which he was posted to 350 Sqn on 23 December 1942. He moved to 349 Sqn on 15 June 1943. He then moved to 18 APC Eastchurch (10 May 1944), 57 OTU Eskett (17 October 1944), 84 GSU Thruxton, 349 Sqn (20 November 1944), 83 GSU Westhampnett (21 December 1944), and finally on 10 January 1945 returned to 350 Sqn then based at Y.32 Ophoven. He was killed in combat on 20 April 1945 during a sweep in the Neuruppin area. His awards included: Knight of the Order of Leopold II with Palm and Belgian Croix de Guerre with Palm. At the time of his death his rank was Warrant Officer. He had only one victory to his credit, that of 2 March 1945.

[14] E. Pauwels (RAF no. 1424929) – apart from the two claims for a damaged and probably destroyed Bf109s, he also claimed two Fw190s destroyed on 25 April 1945.

[15] No P-47 losses are included in USAAF listings. The 9th AF which flew numerous strafing missions in the morning, lost no machines to enemy fighters.

Propellers and jets

Fighter pilots of the 9th AF flew many attacks against ground targets in the morning of 2 March 1945. Some of these resulted in encounters with German jet aircraft.

Thunderbolt pilots of the 365 FG, having just moved from Metz to Florennes/Juzaine aerodrome in Belgium, engaged their old adversaries from KG 51 over north-west Germany. A total of four attacks were performed against the Thunderbolts that strafed targets in the area in the morning. At 10.05 the flight of Lt Archi F. Maltbi from the 388 FS was attacked from behind by three jet fighters. The attack forced the Americans to jettison their bombs and abandon their mission. 10 minutes later one Me

Right:
Onboard gun camera footage of 357 FG Mustang showing attack of the german fighter on B-17 bomber.
via 357 FG Assn.

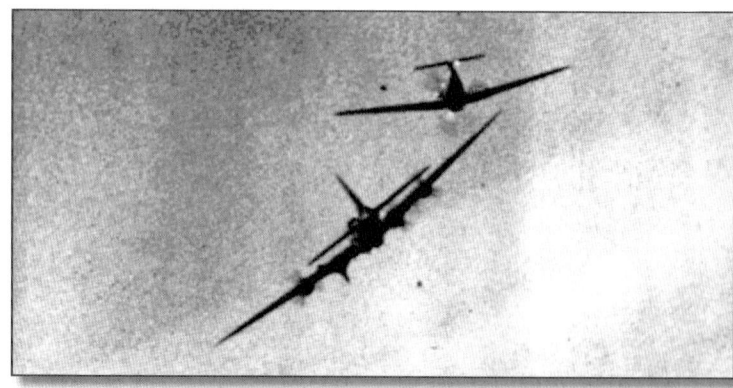

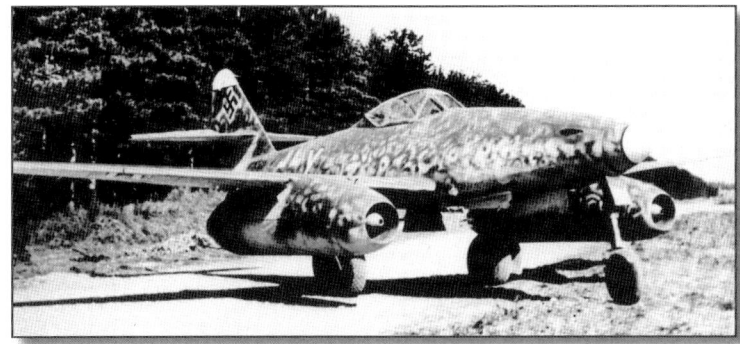

Me 262 A-2a of KG 51
R. Pęczkowski coll.

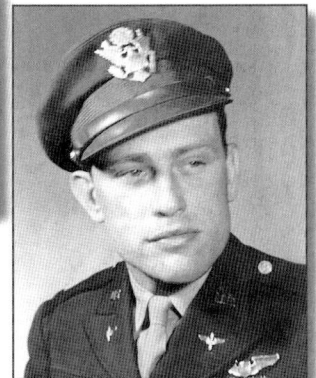

An official portrait picture of Capt. Bruno Peters, 354 FG.
via B. Peters

262 dived to attack the formation led by Capt. Russell L. Gardner from the 387 FS. Following this unsuccessful attack the German pilot used his superior speed to quickly disappear from the scene. At 10.20 the flight of Lt Warren J. Jahnke (387 FS) was on its way back from the target, a factory in Holland. That moment they were came under an unsuccessful attack by a German jet fighter that immediately left the scene, as in the case described above. The fourth encounter of American fighter pilots with German jets took place at 11.05. Lt Robert Rollo re-grouped his flight from the 386 FS after an attack against the railway station at Gladbach, when they spotted two Me 262s flying over Cologne. The German machines were 1200 m below, but they quickly climbed towards the US formation. Rollo gave order to attack, but the Me 262s aborted their attack and turned back. After a few minutes Rollo abandoned the unsuccessful chase which he later described: *'It was like rhinos chasing gazelles'*.

These morning incidents suggest that the German pilots from KG 51 had mastered their machines completely, and having carried out their bombing tasks, they were looking for American fighters as targets of opportunity.

Even with the master skills of the pilots these missions were not without losses. Hptm. Fritz Abel, the CO of 5 Staffel II/KG 51, was killed in his Me 262A-2a W.Nr. 110553 (9K+EN) at Nijmegen. He was shot down by 1/Lt Floyd T. Dunmire of the 107th Recon Sqn flying an F-6 Mustang, who at 10.15 claimed an Me 262 probably destroyed. II/KG 51 lost two more machines when landing at Mühlheim. The Me 262A-2a W.Nr. 110941 forced landed at Mühlheim and was 50% damaged. The other Messerschmitt, Me 262A-2a W.Nr. 110516 (NY+BR), was also forced to land at Mühlheim 20% damaged. Both these accidents were due to pilot error or technical failure.

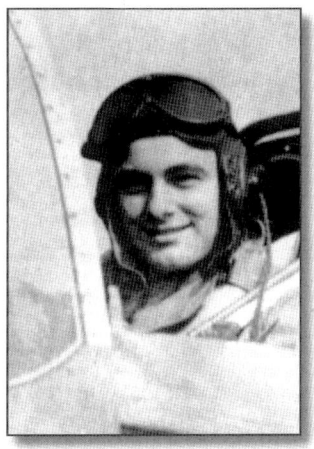

1/Lt. Frederick T. O'Connor, 364 FG, 384 FS claimed one Me 262 as probably shot down.
via Ch. Carter

Encounters between 9th AF Mustangs and Me 262s were also becoming more and more frequent. In the morning Capt. James P. Keane led a formation of 16 P-51s to the Dieburg area. For the 353 FS this was the first operation during March. The fighter sweep resulted in four damaged and one destroyed locomotive and 66 damaged railway cars of various kinds. During the mission, at 09.15 Lt Cary announced over the radio a train south of Dillingen. 1/Lt Theodore W. Sedvert from the 353 FS 354 FG dived in his P-51 to attack the locomotive. But as soon as he emerged from clouds, much to his surprise he saw an Me 262 flying ahead and below. From his superior height he held behind the enemy and with one three-second burst hit the Messerschmitt's fuselage, starboard engine, and cockpit area. The pilot of the Messerschmitt dropped his canopy, but due to the low altitude the German pilot was not able to bale out. He decided to force-land, but upon touch-down the damaged machine exploded, killing the pilot. On 2 March 1945 the Luftwaffe lost in that area Me 262A-1a W.Nr.110655 from I/EKG(J) 1, and its pilot Ofhr. Horst Metzbrand was killed. It seems certain that it was Ofhr. Metzbrand who fell prey to Lt Sedvert. The leader of the sweep, Capt. James P. Keane, claimed destruction of a German Fw 44 at 10.00 in the area of Illesheim aerodrome. German records mentioned the loss of the Fw44 W.Nr.2953 from I/EKG (J), but the name and fate of the pilot is not known.

More Messerschmitt 262s destroyed were claimed by pilots of the 354 FG. Capt. Bruno Peters led a sweep of the 355 FS in the area of Fulda and south of Kassel:

'I was the leader of two flights of P51s, four airplanes in each flight. We were on a mission to Seek and Destroy also known as Targets of Opportunity. We used some of our ammo earlier but I can't recall the targets. We were on our way to home base, Toul Rosieres Air Base TRAB. At 10,000 or 12,000 feet above a cloud cover, with some breaks, we passed over an airport. We noted that 4 aircraft were taking off.

I directed one flight to stay up for top cover. I took my flight to engage the 4 'bogies'. In the descent through the clouds, my wingman, Lt Delgado and I ended up right on the tails of what turned out to be Me 262s. With speed built up in the dive, I advised Delgado to attack the #4 aircraft. I moved in on #3. While we are both firing, out of the corner of my eye, I saw the pilot of Lt Delgado's target bail out. My target went into a descent, allowing me to pull up on #2 aircraft and fire upon it, which also went into a descent. About this time the leader spotted a P51 on each side of his Me 262. He poured on the power & our speed was dissipating from the descent. I yelled 'let's get out of here'. I was concerned we hadn't any ammunition left. We received no anti aircraft fire until we left. On return to our base, calculating time & heading from the target, I estimated that we were over Kassel.'

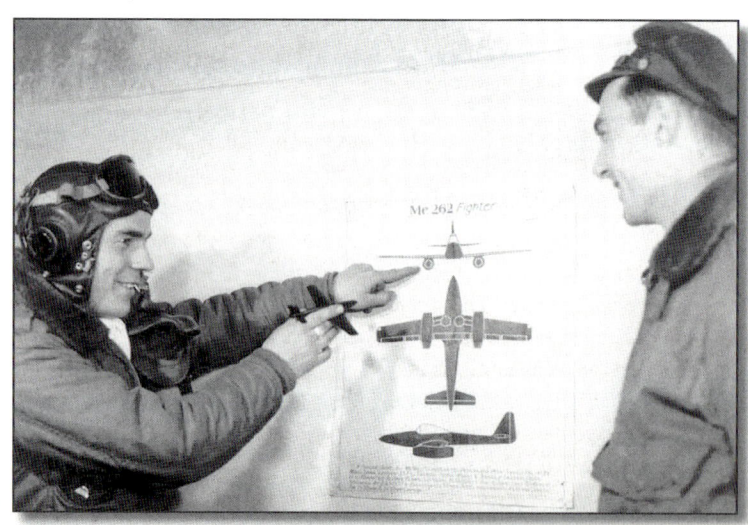

Using a model of a North American P-51 Mustang and a drawing of an Me 262, Flight Officer Ralph Delgado Jr., Milltown, NJ, (left) explains to 2nd Lt. Charles D. Kilpatrick, Newark, NJ, the tactics he used in destroying the twin engine German jet fighter, the 700th enemy plane shot down by his group. Both men are members of the crack 354th Fighter-Bomber Group of the 9th AF, which has also destroyed hundreds of tanks, motor transport, locomotives, & railroad cars.

via B. Peters

Upon return to base Capt. Bruno Peters and F/O Ralph Delgado each claimed one Me 262 damaged, possibly destroyed near Kassel aerodrome. It is true, though, that I/KG (J) 54 lost no less than four Me 262s that day. The rescue group of four Me262s from 3/KG (J) 54 had just taken off from Giebelstadt to attack bombers when they were attacked by Mustangs of the 354 FG. Fhr. Heinrich Griems in Me262 W.Nr.111899 fell to Capt. Peters. Another lost pilot, Fw. Günther Görlitz in Me 262 W.Nr.110913, baled out wounded from his damaged Messerschmitt over Würzburg. He must have been shot down by F/O Delgado. The third lost machine, Me 262 A-1 W.Nr.111887, was flown by Lt. Wolfgang Zimmerman who was killed. It seems quite probable that he was another victim of Capt. Peters during the latter's second attack. There is information about a fourth machine lost, provided by the research group gathered around the *www.stormbirds.com* website. Apparently this was W.Nr.900699, also shot down during take-off by American P-51s.

One Me 262 was claimed as probably destroyed by Lt Fred O´Connor from the 383 FS 364 FG.

'My flight flew at an altitude of 15,000 feet. Then we saw two Me 262s flying west at an altitude of 12,000 feet. We started to chase them, but were unable to catch up with them until they turned east. As we approached, they split. Me and my wingman chased one. I had no problem outmanoeuvring the German machine. Yet, the pilot mastered his machine perfectly and performed wild turns. I fired in turns. After about two minutes he headed down through the clouds. I last saw him in a 70-degree flight downwards at an altitude of 3,000 feet. He trailed white smoke that came out from under the fuselage. I claim one Me 262 probably destroyed 15 km north-east of Frankfurt.' The victory took place at 12.35.

The last action of the Allies against the Me 262s that took place in the afternoon proved favourable for the Germans. A group of Thunderbolts from an unidentified 9th AF unit attacked the aerodrome at Kitzingen, then the base of II/KG(J) 54 under Hptm. Ernst Petzold, where a number of Me 262s gathered after a formation practice flight. In spite of intensive fire from the P-47s none of the Messerschmitts was destroyed or even seriously damaged.

8th AF - Mission 859

This did not, however, end this day, so unlucky for the Luftwaffe. In fact this had started already on 1 March 1945 with information about the weather situation for the following day, intended for the 8th AF HQ. This forecasted favourable weather conditions and good visibility. Based on this information, at 16.00 the 8th AF HQ decided to attack in the Magdeburg area. Should the weather deteriorate, the machines were supposed to try to hit their targets using H2X on-board radars.

38 bomb groups of the 8th Air Force were put on alert in Britain. They had a total of 1,210 four-engined bombers. The machines were organised in three Task Forces.

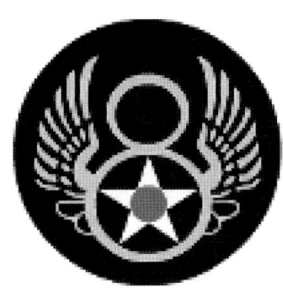

Insignia of the 8th AF.

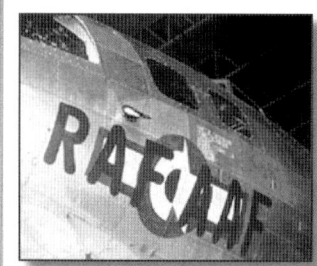

Nose art of B-17G 44-6883 (MS-Q) "RAFAAF", 535 BS, 381 BG, 8 AF.

via 381 BG Assn

Task Force I had 444 B-17 Flying Fortresses of the 1st Air Division. Their targets were the following: 305 BG was going to attack an AA battery situated 10 km south-east of Böhlen. The 306, 92, 398, 91, 381, 457, 351 and 401 BGs were scheduled to attack the synthetic oil plant (old and new works) Braunkohle-Benzin A.G. at Böhlen, while the 384, 379 and 303 BGs were to attack the Rositz oil refinery.

Task Force II had 445 B-17 Flying Fortresses of the 3rd Air Division. Their targets were as follows: the 385, 34, 490, 390, 100, 95, 388 and 96 BGs were going to attack the synthetic oil plant Braunkohle-Benzin A.G. at Schwarzheide, while the 487, 447, 94 and 486 BGs were going to strike at the jet aircraft assembly plant at Alt-Lonnewitz.

Task Force III had 321 B-24 Liberators of the 2nd Air Division. The 491, 392, and 446 BGs were planned to attack the synthetic oil plant of Braunkohle-Benzin A.G. at Magdeburg/Rothensee. The 453, 389, 445, 491, 44, 392, 448, 93, 458, 467 and 466 BGs were going to bomb the tank and armament works at Magdeburg/Buckau, and the oil equipment and torpedo components works at Magdeburg/Buckau.

After detailed planning and assignment of tasks, Mission no. 859 could finally begin.

Task Force I

Four-engined bombers of the 12 bomb groups took off from the 8th AF aerodromes at 06.00-06.40 and, grouped in Task Force I, crossed the Channel, heading for France and the southern Ruhr, towards Böhlen. Fighter escort for Task Force I consisted of 273 Mustangs of five fighter groups: 54 aircraft from the 20 FG, 62 from the 352 FG, 57 from the 356 FG, 46 from the 359 FG and 54 machines from the 364 FG. Some of these were forced to turn back due to various failures, so eventually some 260 P-51 fighters were going to defend their 'big friends'. They flew ahead of the attacking formation and patrolled the area around the river Rhine and the city of Frankfurt.

In the target area Task Force I met unfavourable weather conditions, 8/10th cloud cover made up of cumulus and stratocumulus, with the top at 8,000-10,000 feet (2,400-3,000 m). Most crews were not able to bomb their primary target, but more attention was paid to the secondary target, the city of Chemnitz. The entire attack was carried out using the H2X guidance system.

The AA battery at Böhlen was attacked by the 305 BG from an altitude of 23,400-24,500 feet (7,100-7,500 m). Between 10.36 and 10.42, 36 Flying Fortresses dropped their bombs. A nearby ammunition dump was also hit.

The primary target at Böhlen was attacked by the full complement of the 92 BG, led by Maj. John R. McKee, together with the 306(A) and 306(B) BGs. Between 10.45 and 10.53, 60 B-17s dropped their loads from an altitude of 23,600-26,000 feet (7,200-7,900 m). Post-raid photos showed the extent of damage. At least 70 hits on target, with direct hits in the most important areas of the factory. Also the Sachsische Werke power station was seriously damaged.

Of the three groups initially intended for Rositz, only the 384 BG attacked it. 37 aircraft dropped their bombs from an altitude of 25,800-26,800 feet (7,900-8,200 m). The attack commenced at 11.00 and continued for 7 minutes. Bombs fell on the central and north-west part of the complex.

The secondary target was attacked by most machines of Task Force I. This was the marshalling yard at Chemnitz. The 250 four-engined bombers dropped 3,440 bombs. The first bombs left the bomb bays of the Fortresses at 10.17, and the sirens did not stop screaming until 11.04, when the last Fortress dropped its war load. Due to clouds over target the H2X system was used, and no precise photos could be taken after the raid. On those that were 'legible', one could see just 250 bomb craters. Some bombs fell on the main railway station, destroying it, some fell on the fields and villages 4 miles (6 km) south-east of Chemnitz. A group of bombs fell on an unidentified factory 4 miles (6 km) south-south west of the station. 253 people, including some children, were killed during the attack on the city.

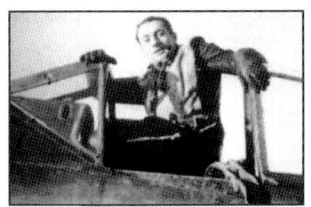

Ofw. Hans Todt, 8. JG 301.
via Reschke

The 381 BG was one of those groups that attacked Chemnitz. Its 37 aircraft, led by Capt. Tyson, dropped their bombs on the target. This bomb group had an interesting experience that day. Upon take-off Lt Charles 'Hotrock' Carpenter had an engine failure and returned in his B-17. Col. Shackley from the control tower called him back to land. Carpenter landed smoothly in his fully loaded and fuelled Fort. His crew quickly moved to another aircraft and took off. They were some 20 minutes behind their main formation, so Carpenter opened up to try to catch the other bombers. While screening the sky he saw a large number of aircraft far away. He picked up speed and got closer. To his surprise they were British Lancasters. It was too late to change his mind, so he joined the Lancasters to their target, Cologne on the Rhine (see Annex). Lt Carpenter dropped his bombs together with the RAF aircraft. It was only after the bombs were gone that the Lancaster crews noticed him. Gun turrets of the Lancasters turned towards the lone Fortress in the formation, and strange conversation could be heard over the radio. Once all was clarified, Carpenter picked two Lancasters as wingmen, and went home. Upon landing Lt Carpenter realised that his bomber was named 'RAFAAF', a combination of the Royal Air Force and Army Air Forces acronyms…

Another unit that attacked Chemnitz was the 401 BG. The last of the 39 machines led by Maj. C. A. Lewis took off from Deenethorpe at 07.07. Having pointed out to the Mustang pilots that the primary target was covered with clouds, the group decided to attack the secondary target, Chemnitz. The attack was carried out without problems and all machines returned safely to Britain.

The rest of Task Force I dropped its bombs on targets of opportunity: Saalfeld, Kaaden (Kadaň in Czechoslovakia), Penig, and the railway bridge at Jocket. Saalfeld was attacked at 11.29 by bombers of the 398(B) BG. 13 bombers dropped 29.2 tonnes of bombs on the town from an altitude of 25,300 feet (7,700 m). The rail bridge at Jocket was 'visited' by 11 bombers from the 91(C) BG. At 11.06 these dropped 24.6 tonnes of bombs from an altitude of 24,590 feet (7,500 m). 65 bombs exploded on the bridge or near it. The station at Penig was attacked by 12 B-17s that dropped 25.8 tonnes of bombs. Approximately 100 hits observed on the rail tracks rendered the line useless. According to American records, bombs on Kaaden were dropped from an altitude of 20,000 feet at 11.04 by 11 B-17s from the 398(C) BG.

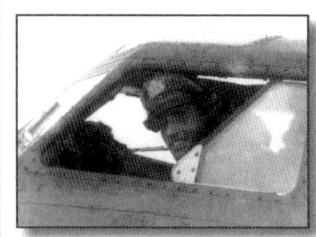

2/Lt. Donald R. Christensen (KIA), 398 BG, 603 BS. Pilot of a B-17 which crashed near the Czech village of Slany.

via J. Kohout

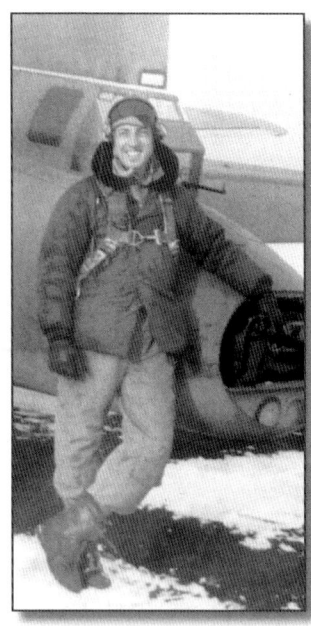

Sgt. Selmer K. Haakenson - tail gunner. The only airman who survived the attack by Fw 190s and described the fate of his fellow crew members.

via J. Kohout

[16] *From J. Kohout publication, courtesy of the author.*

However, no bombs fell on Kadaň that day. On the other hand, Ústí nad Labem (Aussig) was 'visited' by a few American bombers which placed their war load there. That raid was not mentioned in American records, so probably this was a case of misidentification, and the Americans mistook Ústí nad Labem for Kadaň. A river runs through each of the towns...

Bomber units lost three aircraft. The 305 BG lost two machines (B-17G 44-8141 from the 365 BS and B-17G 43-38102 from the 366 BS), one of which was downed by Flak. The third bomber lost belonged to the 603 BS 398 BG. The Boeing B-17G 44-6573 (ET-K) of 2/Lt Donald R. Christensen fell prey to one of six enemy fighters, probably from II Gruppe JG 301.

The rear turret of the bomber was manned by Sgt Selmer K. Haakeson:

'Some 30 minutes prior to arrival over the target we were forced to jettison two bombs due to aileron problems. The flight engineer, upper gunner Sgt Robert W. Dudley, went to move the ailerons up using a crank. Shortly after his return we were attacked by some six Fw190s and we received some hits. One shot put out my intercom. Shrapnel hit me on the right hand side of my face, so that I could barely see. The blow threw me backwards on the floor. I grabbed the parachute and attached it by a single belt to the equipment. I returned to my place and continued to fire.

Then the rear portion detached from the damaged fuselage and spun down with me. Because of the enormous force acting there I was unable to bale out. About 1,200 m over the ground falling became smoother, and I was able to shed my bullet-proof vest, attach my parachute properly, and bale out through the rear door'.

The rear portion of the bomber fell near Pchery. Having baled out of the B-17's tail over the valley of Theodor, Sgt Haakeson landed with his parachute over the northern edge of Olšany. Heavily wounded, the airman landed near the last buildings of the settlement. Upon landing he was arrested by Czech Protectorate guards from the Brandýsk post. He was given first-aid and then taken by a military ambulance to the hospital at Slany.

The heavily damaged bomber fell rapidly to the ground, taking with it the other eight airmen. The B-17 crashed about 11.00 on the 'Na tehuli' field not far from Kvíč. All the eight men were killed in the wreckage. Their remains were taken to the cemetery at Slany and buried with all honours after the intervention of the International Red Cross. The wreckage was removed in March 1945.[16]

The only fighter of II Gruppe JG 301 who claimed a bomber shot down that day was Oberfeldweber Hans Todt of 8 Staffel JG 301. Therefore, it seems he may have downed the crew of Christensen.

Other bombers, damaged by German fighters, were forced to land on the Allied side of the continent. These included the B-17 43-38858 from the 327 BS 92 BG. 54 aircraft returned to base damaged by Flak. One crew member was killed, four were wounded, and 29 were declared Missing in Action.

Bombers of Task Force I dropped 1,015 tonnes of bombs on their targets. Out of this number 310 tonnes dropped by 133 aircraft fell on primary targets, 250 bombers dropped 593.6 tonnes of bombs on secondary targets, and 50 aircraft dropped 111.8 tonnes of bombs on targets of opportunity.

The operational day ended for Task Force I between 15.00 and 16.30, when last bombers of the 1st Air Division alighted on the grass strips of England.

Task Force I fighter escort

Task Force I was not attacked by any numerous Luftwaffe units. The enemy appeared in the air sporadically and in small formations. In case of a major grouping of enemy fighters the fighter escort was on alert and forced the enemy to retreat with serious losses.

One fighter group, before it turned for the secondary target between Böhlen and Rositz, spotted three Fw190s. South of Chemnitz five single-seat enemy fighters were seen, but German pilots did not attack.

Upon return to their bases American fighter pilots claimed 8-1-4(6)[17] victories.

Two damaged Fw 190s were claimed by pilots of the 20 FG upon return from their Mission no. 272.

The 20 FG, led by Maj. Meyer (A Group) and Maj. Gatterdam (B Group) took off at 07.45 and at 09.30 rendezvoused with the bombers northwest of Frankfurt. After the bombardment the formation was attacked by some 6 Fw190s and two Bf 109s. The 77 FS engaged the German fighters. American fighter pilots managed to break the attack against the B-17s, but one of the Fw 190 pilots managed to score a hit.

Lt David F. McCalister[18] chased one Focke Wulf in a dive down to 15,000 feet (5,000 m). He fired several bursts into it. Then he returned to the bombers. The Fw 190 that he chased was last seen spinning towards the ground. Lt Reps D. Jones 'hovered' behind the other Focke Wulf and started to chase it. At an altitude of 6,000 feet (2,000 m) he fired several times at the German. He was not able to see the results of his fire, as the German machine disappeared in clouds below. Both claimed their Fw 190s as damaged.

Other victories were scored by pilots of the 352 FG who claimed 8-0-2(6) victories. The 328 FS took off at 08.32, and the 487 FS at 08.40. They probably engaged pilots of I Gruppe JG 301 'Wilde Sau', who had taken off from Salzwedel, and of II/JG 301 'Wilde Sau' from Stendal. Pilots of the 486 FS bounced 16 Fw190A-9s and 'long-nose' Fw 190D-9s that attempted to attack the bombers. German pilots attacked four machines in

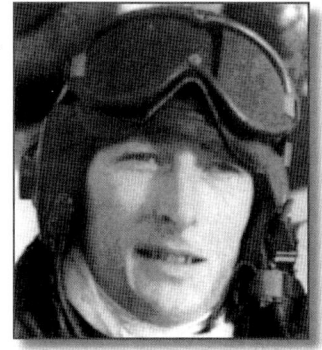

2/Lt. David F. "Mac" McCallister - total WWII score = 1 FW 190 damaged.

20 FG Assn.

Above Left:
Wreck of the B-17 near village Slany.

via J. Kohout

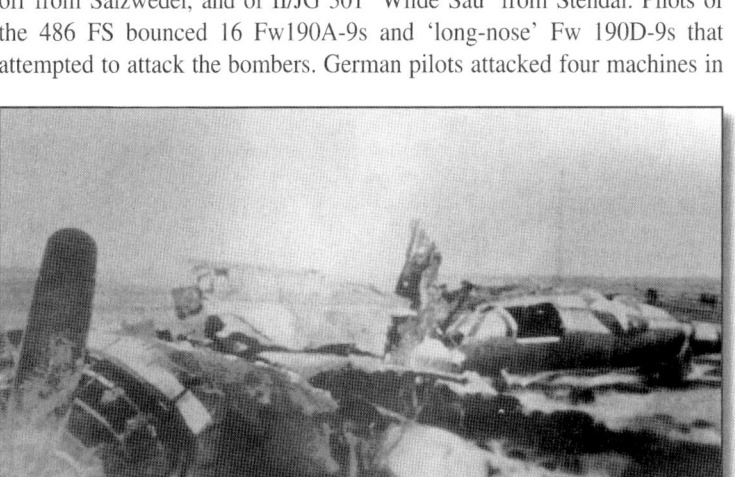

[17] American system of victory classification: destroyed-damaged-probable. Aircraft destroyed on the ground are included in brackets.

[18] David Franklin McCallister. Born February 02, 1920; Died June 04, 1961. He is buried at Arlington National Cemetery: Section 30 Site 2131

An Ordinary Day in 1945

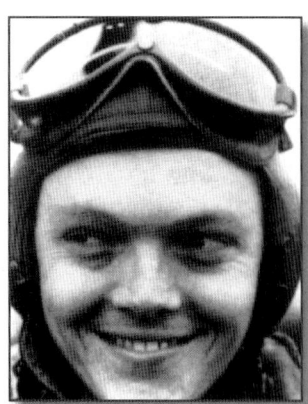

Capt. Reps D. Jones - total WWII score 2-1-1 (5-0-1).
20 FG Assn.

the top squadron of the 398 BG from above, out of the sun. Although they undertook just one attack, the fighter escort of the bombers wasted no time and between 10.45 and 11.10 American fighter pilots claimed destruction or damage to seven Fw 190s in the area of Prague, Zwickau, Zwebau, and Chemnitz. Captain Edwin L. Heller, the Squadron CO, shot down one German machine, and damaged another Fw 190.

'I headed north from the target as there were more bombers up there. As I approached them, I noticed fifteen plus bogies coming in from the right. Just then they nosed over and went through a box of bombers. I dropped tanks and told my squadron we would attack.

I tried to bounce the last of them, but the leading flight turned into me, so I in turn turned into them. There ensued a Luftbery of all planes. The fight was underway only a few minutes when I noticed at least six Fw 190s burning or spinning down. At one time during the scrap, lining up on one enemy aircraft, I glanced back to clear my tail, and saw a 190 queuing up on me. At that instant he burst into flames, as my wingman, Lt Paulson, got him in the sights before he could get a shot at me.

I got some hits on my 190, but as it was a 90 degree deflection shot, I only damaged him. There were more 190s in the sky so I let him go and got on another Hun's tail. He was pulling up behind a box of bombers when I closed on him. I got many hits in the cockpit and a lot of pieces came off. I am sure I killed him as the plane went down out of control. I looked around for another fight, but there weren't any Jerry planes left.'

Three pilots of I/JG 301 were killed in the encounter, and one baled out. Things were worse with II/JG 301. Seven pilots lost their lives and three machines were destroyed without loss of pilots. Survivors of the combat with the Americans included Fj.Uffz. Helmut-Peter Rix[19] of 8 Staffel. His account provides insight into the encounter from the German pilot's viewpoint:

'Our schwarm took off at 10.15 from Stendal, to stop the American raid. We were led by Staffelkapitän Lt. Walter Kropp in a D-9. I flew Fw 190D-9 'red 4'[20]. Two more pilots of our schwarm, Uffz. Heger and Uffz. Ehrlich, flew in Fw 190A-9s.

This was my first combat sortie. We climbed to 24,000 feet (7,300 m). Then we spotted, some 3,000 feet (1,000 m) above, formations of B-17s. Our schwarm leader made a climbing turn to port. I followed. As no. 4 I was outboard. It was a beautiful morning with clear sky, with clouds at 14,000 feet (4,300 m) below.

Once we broke through the clouds, I felt a jolt in my machine, and the engine stopped working smoothly. Flames appeared and rose. It was unbearably hot in the cockpit, so I had to bale out. I jettisoned the canopy, and could only watch my aircraft, as it fell to the ground out of control. I saw no other enemy aircraft, even Flak did not fire. I did not know how all this had happened. Upon landing in snow I realised I had several wounds on my head, face, and arm. I could barely see due to the head wounds. Fortunately a local farmer ran to the spot where I landed, and he took me to the hospital at Aussig (Ústí nad Labem in the Czech Republic – author's note)'.

In fact, Rix was given initial medical examination by Dr Sasyn from Petrovice. Then, until 14.00, the German pilot stayed at the estate of

[19] Lt. Helmut Peter Rix was born in 1924 in a village near Krefeld. After graduating as a pilot, he was sent to I/JG 2 for more training. On 12 January 1945 he was posted to 8. Staffel of II/JG 301 at Welzow, but did not see combat until 2 March 1945. He was shot down in his first combat mission.

[20] The Fw 190D-9s flown by Kropp and Rix were most probably both borrowed from 6 Staffel. This is based on the red marking (6 Staffel used red colours and type of aircraft (8. Staffel) was equipped with the Fw 190A-9). W.Nr.500111, flown by Rix, has also been reported 10% damaged on 1 January 1945 during Operation 'Bo-denplatte' as an aircraft of 3/JG 2 flolwn by Uffz. Herbert Körber (WIA), who landed at Merzhausen.

Gertruda Zechelova at Větrov, until Wehrmacht soldiers took him to the hospital at Ústí nad Labem. Rix returned to his unit on 20 April, but doctors did not allow him to fly any more. When Rix was shot down, his machine crashed at 10.40 some 600 m from Kratzhammer village on the Saxon side of the border, 4 km north of Větrov. Soon before that the pilot was seen to bale out from the burning aircraft and fall towards Větrov. The abandoned machine exploded at an altitude of some 3,000 m. Rix was the only survivor of the schwarm led by Lt. Kropp. Exact identification of his victor is not possible, but it is probably that he was shot down by one of two pilots of the 486 FS 352 FG: Capt. Lee E. Kilgo or 1/Lt Earl L. Mundel, who claimed Fw 190s destroyed at 11.00.

In his Combat Report, Kilgo wrote: *'I was flying No. 4 in yellow flight when the flight engaged one Fw 190 and began a Luftbery. The enemy aircraft turned away, placing me in position on his tail. At long range I fired several bursts and he began smoking and went into a turning dive directly over a town. I broke away – the flight leader saw him crash in flames'*

Capt. Edwin L. Heller, 352 FG.
352 FG Assn.

The other possible victor of Peter Rix is Earl Mundel. *'My flight was higher, thereby giving me a better chance to close on him. I was making good progress when two P-51s came in from the side. One ship got several hits. The 190 threw to an altitude of 15 000 feet. I tacked on, fired a long burst, – some parts fell off and the pilot bailed out near 8 000 feet. The ship hit and exploded not far from a small town.'*

Having successfully defended the bombers, 352 FG pilots, and to be exact the section led by Lt Col. Willie Jackson, descended to the ground, to look for Luftwaffe aerodromes or other targets of opportunity, to spend their ammunition. One of their targets was the aerodrome at Prague-Ruzyň.

'I was leading B-Group when a few enemy aircraft were seen to dive through the bombers in the target area. We dropped our tanks and gave chase to the deck, ending up at the airfield west of Prague. We engaged an Fw 190 at 17 000 feet over the drome and I fired a couple of bursts at him but got no strikes. Captain Kilgo and Lt Mundell cut in and clobbered him. The pilot hit the silk and the plane crashed. (It was the action reported above, where Lt. Rix was shot down – author's note)

I then made a dive-strafing attack on the field to check the Flak. After pulling up I observed an enemy aircraft taking off which I identified as

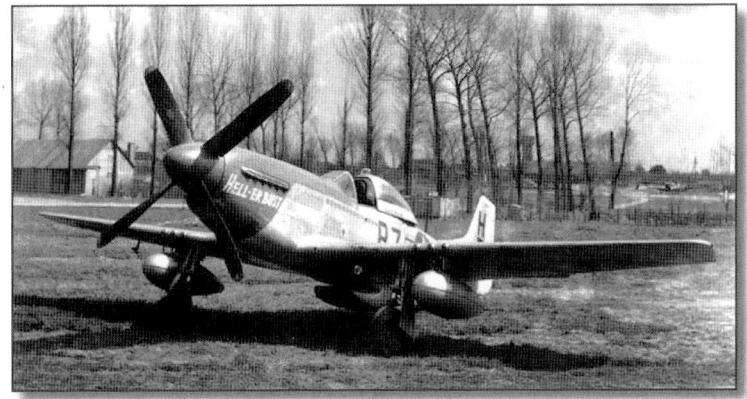

Left:
"Hell-Er Burst". Personal plane of Capt. Edwin L. Heller, 352 FG.
352 FG Assn.

Official report of Helmut - Peter Rix.

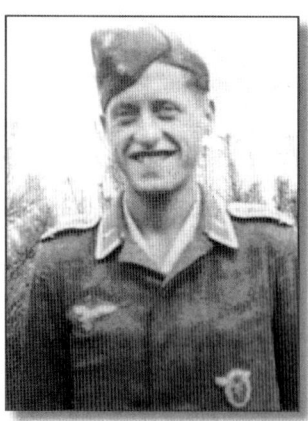

Only survivor of the Schwarm led by Lt. Kropp. FUffz. Helmut - Peter Rix, 8./ JG 301.
via H.P.Rix

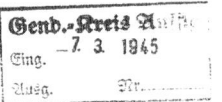

an Fw 189. I spiralled down and closed rapidly on him as he turned back toward the field possibly to lure us over the Flak positions. I opened fire and saw my fire hitting behind him so I pulled my lead in and got a concentration of good strikes in the cockpit and engines. Pieces flew off and the enemy aircraft started trailing smoke and flames. The pilot was either dead or badly hit. The enemy aircraft crashed about half a mile north-east of the field. It happened at 11.15.'

The Luftwaffe lost no machine of the type, or at least no trace of such loss was left in the records.

Apart from the Fw 189, Lt Col. Jackson claimed two unidentified twin-engined aircraft as damaged at the aerodrome. Four more damaged aircraft were claimed (two each) by Capt. Chet Harker and Lt C.C. Pattillo[21]. The group flew over the aerodrome no less than six times before powerful Flak came into action. Then the Americans left the place.

Damage to German machines must have been minimal, as no information on the strafing was recorded.

Task Force II

Between 06.20 and 07.10 Flying Fortresses of twelve 8th AF groups took off from their bases and formed Task Force II. Together with aircraft of Task Force III they crossed the Channel and Dutch coast, heading for Brunswick. Task Force II led the way. Once over the continent, the 'big

[21] *Pattillo claimed destruction of five enemy machines, but only two were credited.*

buddies' were joined by their fighter escort - 231 Mustangs from five fighter groups were to ensure a safe flight. Bombers of Task Force II were going to penetrate the furthest inland, so a German attack was expected against these bombers. Before the story moves on to how these expectations were verified, the raid itself will be described.

Above the target clouds appeared at an altitude of 8,000-10,000 feet (2,500-3,000 m). Visibility was almost nil, with 8/10 cloud cover over the target.

The primary target, the synthetic oil plant of Braunkohle-Benzin A.G., was bombed at 10.31 from an altitude of 22,500 feet (6,900 m) by two groups. 24 B-17s from the 95(A) and 95(C) BG dropped their bombs using the H2X homing system. Photos taken on 3 March proved the bombing was effective. The south-east part of the complex was hit by a group of bombs. A neighbouring village was also hit several times. The south-east part of the factory complex was hit by the second 'series' of bombs which damaged or completely destroyed the objective. However, after overall evaluation, the effects of the attack were not considered good in terms of stopping the work of the plant. The parts that were hit were not important enough to stop production completely.

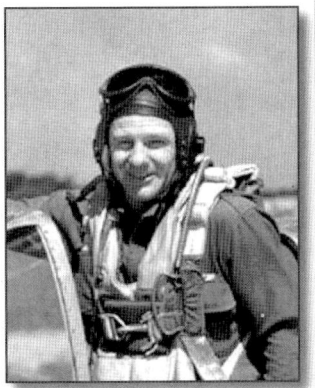

1/Lt. Earl L. Mundel, 352 FG.
352 FG Assn.

The secondary target at Dresden was attacked by a majority of the Task Force II bombers. 402 B-17s dropped their lethal cargo from an altitude of 18,750-23,900 feet (5,700-7,300 m) between 10.27 and 11.07 on the marshalling yard. However, most of the 'greetings' fell some half a mile (800 m) north of the planned point of the attack, so in fact this raid proved a complete failure. Still, the 'Mighty Eighth' and the RAF had already visited the target several times, so the crews of the bombers may have seen scenes of destruction in the city below. The 34 BG was attacked by fighters and that was why it failed to hit accurately. The centre of the city was marked as the hit area. A formation of 38 bombers from the 34 BG was led by Col. Young. Their crews dropped 92.25 tonnes of bombs on the town. In spite of the attack by German fighters the 34 BG recorded no losses to them. In the B-17G 44-8670 flown by Lt Z. C. Richardson one crew member was killed: S/Sgt John H. Frey from Cincinnati, Ohio, a waist gunner.

34 BG gunners claimed 3-7-2 victories:

Gunner	Post	Aircraft	BS	Pilot	Claim
Robinson	W/G	43-38380	391	Sherman	1 destroyed
Archer	B/T	43-38257	391	Wilcox	1 damaged
Allen	TTG	43-38991	18	W.S. Jones	1 destroyed
Reo	W/G	44-8605	18	Abrams	1 damaged
Roe	TTG	44-6938	18	Nass	1 destroyed
Lombard	TTG	43-38216	18	Kennedy	1 damaged
Johnson	T/G	43-38386	7	Rocher	1 damaged
Graham	T/G	44-8309	7	R. Martin	1 damaged
Alexander	TTG	44-6296	7	Wright	1 damaged
McArdle	T/G	43-38334	7	Hicks	1 probably destroyed
Wyder	W/G	43-38416	7	O'Grady	1 damaged
Reed	B/T	43-38280	7	MacTaggart	1 probably destroyed

Photos of the 447 BG show that bombs fell on the residential district of Dresden-Übigau, some 3.5 km away from the nearest railway building. Considering the type of bombs, bomber crews maintained that the aim was to destroy the city completely, or whatever was left of it.

Eight bombers were lost during the mission, and 62 were damaged. Out of the eight machines lost in combat, three bombers were from the 96 BG. Two of these from the 96 BG collided over the Channel at an altitude of 9,000 feet (2,700 m), 10 miles (16 km) south of Southampton. These were B-17G 43-37767 'My Ideal' from the 339 BS and B-17G 44-8697 from the 413 BS.

The incident was recalled by Lt Marty Clayman: '*The lower section was led by Lt Benton Gatch, 339 Squadron, in 43-37767. No. 6 was dangerously close to us. I moved the stick rapidly left and up. The same moment Lt Gatch saw the danger to which his wingman exposed us. Absorbed by the situation, he must have taken his hands off the controls, or pulled them in an unexplained way. The machine lifted and flew upwards. No. 4, Lt Herb Stillwell from the 413 Squadron in 44-8697, flying at the top, cut the climbing leader's machine right aft of the rear turret. Lt Gatch's machine broke in two pieces and fell down. Stillwell's bomber had no nose. Suddenly both his wings detached and the machine fell down irrevocably. I saw one parachute. At the order of the commander I left the formation and circled the spot of the tragedy until the rescue team arrived.*'

None of the eighteen men survived...

Flak over Minden hit the B-17G 43-38828 of 2/Lt William A. Hemphill from the 413 BS 96 BG. The port wing was hit the most. The machine fell from the formation, and it was last seen gliding under control. The bomber crashed near Besterod, 12 km north-east of Kassel. All the crew members survived to become POWs. Not for long.

385 BG, who were flying their 261st mission under Col. G.Y. Jumper, was hit the hardest. About 10.15, while the group was over the Initial Point, it was attacked by enemy fighters. As the bomber crews had not been warned about the presence of the enemy in the area, the bombers approached the target in squadron formations: 385A and 385 B close side by side, and 385C Low some 2-3 miles (3-4.5 km) behind.

The first attack was unexpected. It was performed by 12 Fw190s and 3 Bf109s, probably from II and I/JG 300. They attacked the bombers in three waves. The first six Fw 190s, followed by another six, attacked from behind,

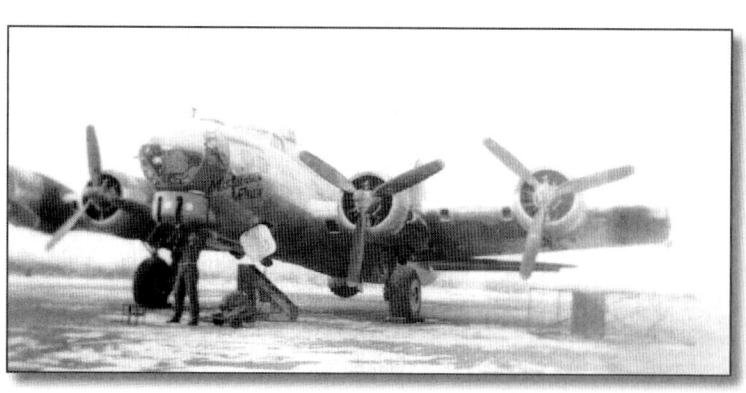

B-17G 43-38280 "Missbehaven Raven", 7 BS, 34 BG, 8 AF. This plane was damaged by flak during the mission. On the other hand, ball turret gunner Reed was one of few gunners who claimed an enemy aircraft probably destroyed.

via G. Ferrell

and after the attack they turned to the port of the formation. Immediately after them, three Messerschmitts attacked from the starboard side. The attack was effective and resulted in the loss of three bombers in positions 3, 5 and 6.

Position no. 3 was Kenneth G. Tipton in B-17G 44-8417 from the 550 BS. The machine was hit near the radio-operator's compartment and in the tail. Engines nos. 1 and 4 started to burn. Controls were half shot away. The tail gunner John Nostin was killed in the crash on the ground, but the other members of the crew survived and spend a short while in captivity. The machine crashed near Fictenburg.

Leon E. Tripp in B-17G 43-38148 from the 549 BS flew as no. 5 in the formation. When the bomber was hit, only the co-pilot, Lt Edward L.C. Batz managed to bale out and was taken prisoner. The bomber crashed near Jüledorf killing the other crew members.

No. 6 was B-17G 42-97979 from the 550 BS flown by Eugene J. Vaadi, with Neil G. Duell as the upper gunner: *'When we started to burn, I remember looking to check the waist and rear gunners. Tony, our engineer, and I checked the fire. The navigator had already left the ship, and we also baled out, seeing how much we were on fire. During the free fall I could see our Fortress 'Leading Lady' explode. I landed directly on the aerodrome of the fighters that were landing at the time. As I touched down strong wind threw me against the ground and I hit myself bad. I could not move for almost a month'.*

The ventral gunner, Jino O. DiFonzo, broke his ankle during the bale out, but all the members of the crew survived the loss of their bomber and became German prisoners.

Enemy aircraft re-formed for another attack. It seemed that they would attack the formation of 385A and B, but they flew over the machines of this close formation and attacked head on the Low squadron in groups of 3 or 4 aircraft. The second attack sealed the fate of B-17G 43-37871 from the 551 BS, flown by 1/Lt Robert Krahn. This was his 30th mission. Krahn recalled how he was shot down: *'We heard on the radio that the Low squadron was attacked by enemy fighters. Next thing that I noticed was that all the Mustangs of the escort turned back to chase the enemy. The first sign of problems came immediately, when the upper gunner Flem Williams started*

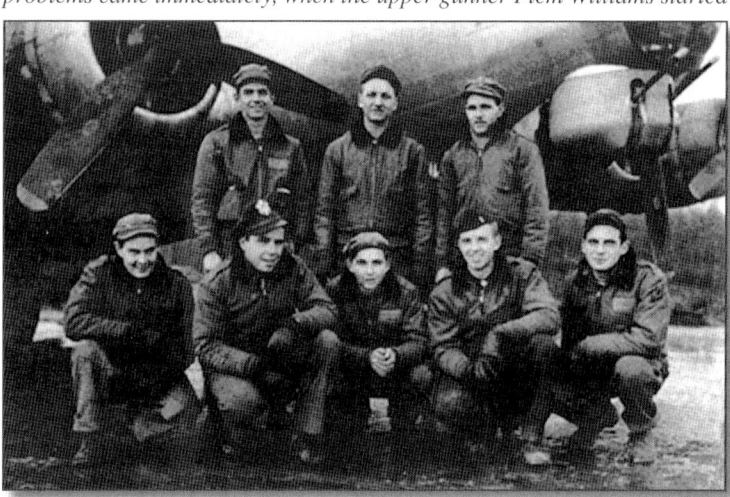

Left:
Crew of Lt. Alberts. Standing (left to right): F.Davitt, L. Eickert, D. Hood; kneeling: A. Stevens, D. Alberts, D. Laubenstine, G. Hale, T. Leone.

390th Memorial Museum Foundation

Right:
B-17G flown by Alberts crew on March 2, 1945.
390th Memorial Museum Foundation

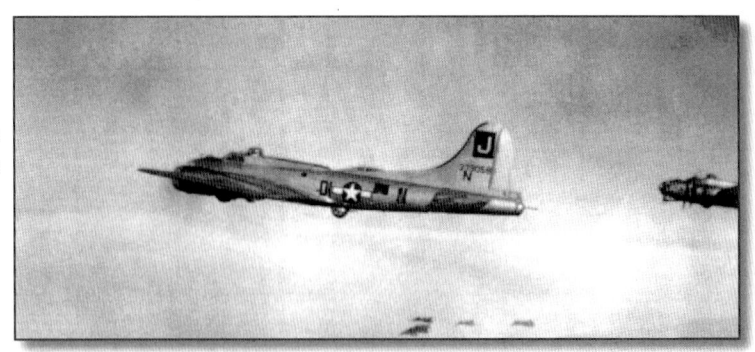

firing at the sun. In a moment 15 Fw 190s in three rows of five machines each bounced us and attacked our formation. I tracked one Fw 190 that flew to my left. The fighter pilot saluted me, and I replied to that instinctively. Then my co-pilot roused me from my thoughts crying: 'We're on fire!' Engine no. 3 was in flames. I kept in formation until we dropped the bombs. After I evaluated the situation, I decided to continue east and land behind Russian lines. I flew diving slightly, hoping that the fire does not spread. That moment the undercarriage dropped and flaps extended due to failure of the electric system. I ordered "abandon ship".

I recall that the Focke Wulf that flew alongside was not grey, as recalled by other airmen, but it was in tan camouflage'.[22]

The pilotless machine crashed on the road between Mimoň and Hradčany, some 100 m north of Hradčany (Česká Lípa district). All nine crew members of 1/Lt Robert A. Krahn's aircraft baled out safely and became POWs. A part of the crew landed at Heřmanovice and Vitkovo.

Then the Mustang escort came to the rescue and the Germans failed to carry out their third attack. Even though they attacked bombers individually, they inflicted no further losses.

The last loss of that formation was from the 390 Bomb Group. At 10.32 B-17G 43-39058 (DI-N) from the 570 Bomb Squadron, flown by 2/Lt Richard A. Alberts was hit by Flak at an altitude of 24,000 feet (7,300 m). The machine was hit in engine no. 3 which started to pour out thick dark smoke, and the bomber left formation and lost height. The pilot turned left and headed for Soviet lines. The group leader was informed by the pilot that the damaged machine was under control and that they expected to reach Soviet lines. That was why nobody baled out. It ended well, when all nine crew members landed safely at Turek near Konin in Poland. All the airmen were escorted to the Soviet military hospital in the city of Łódź, even though only the waist gunner Sgt Mark Warren was wounded.

This was not the only damaged Fortress from the 390 BG. During the flight to the target 43-37565 flown by Lawrence E.W. Roberts collided with 43-38521 flown by Winifred E. Combsom. Both crews managed to get back safely to base, and only one man was wounded: George A. Lockhart from the former machine.

Flak damaged 40 more machines, while enemy fighter pilots 'took care' of four bombers, and damaged seven. Some were forced to land at Melville in France, this being the emergency airfield, code named B-53.

---

[22] This could refer to Fw 190s from JGr.10, as the equip-ment of that training unit was indeed mixed, and the machines may have been still in the camouflage from their previous combat area. The unit probably attacked together with II/JG 300.

One bomber of Task Force II was lost for no known cause. One crew member was killed, two were wounded, and 72 were posted missing in action.

To complete the story of the Task Force II raid, it has to be said that a total of 1,141 tonnes of bombs were dropped by 247 B-17s. 57.9 tonnes fell on the primary target, and 1,081 tonnes on the secondary target. One aircraft dropped its 2.5 tonnes on a target of opportunity.

Task Force II fighter escort

As mentioned before, aircraft of Task Force II flew deepest into Germany that day. No wonder, then, that virtually all the attention of the Luftwaffe focused on these bombers. The fighter escort consisting of five Mustang groups [23] had a lot to do to repel attacks of German Reichsverteidigung (Reich's Defence) fighters. To counter the bombers the Reich Defenders sent some 200 Messerschmitt Bf 109 and Focke Wulf Fw 190 fighters from the 'Wilde Sau' units: JG 300, JG 301 and Jagdgruppe 10 (JGr.10).

About 10.00 the first air combats commenced. More or less half way between Berlin and Magdeburg fighter pilots of the 83 FS 78 FG, flying at the head of the bomber formation, spotted enemy fighters. Col. Landers, who was leading the formation and the entire 78 FG, immediately ordered to attack the Huns. The Germans were probably just assembling their combat formation. 24 Messerschmitts still had their drop tanks attached. The Americans arrived from up sun and started to shoot down one Messerschmitt after another. Pilots at the head of the German formation immediately dropped their external tanks and started to turn rapidly. The remaining machines did not jettison their 300-litre loads, but followed their leaders blindly. Pilots of the German fighters were from IV Gruppe JG 301 'Hindenburg' [24] from Stendal aerodrome, the unit undergoing its baptism of fire that day (the same day the Gruppe moved to Gardelegen). It had been formed only recently, which explained the incompetence of the young and inexperienced pilots. According to American fighters, as soon as they started to be chased, they baled out of their aircraft. Some, however, tried to engage the superior numbers of American fighters. Their pointless efforts ended, in the best case, under a parachute canopy. This happened to Fhr. Blechsmidt and Uffz. Hornschuh, both of 15/JG 301, who baled out wounded from their Messerschmitt Bf 109G-10s over Burg. IV/JG 301 lost 19 aircraft in the encounter with American fighters, this number including landing accidents due to combat damage. Twelve pilots were lost or wounded. The Staffelkapitän 13/JG 301, Oblt. Johan Patek (born on 20 May 1915), was killed in combat.

Later on the engagement was joined by 339 FG, together with the 353 and 357 FGs. On the German side, II, III and IV/JG 300 operating from Löbnitz, Jüterborg-Waldlager and Reinsdorf near Berlin attempted to attack the bombers, and engaged American fighter escorts. This way a major melee started in the triangle of Magdeburg-Berlin-Dresden, dominated by machines with a white star in blue circle.

31 Fw 190A-8 and A-9 aircraft of II/JG 300 attacked the B-17s near Torgau. Their efforts resulted in four bombers from the 385 BG shot down, plus seven more damaged. German pilots claimed five bombers destroyed,

[23] *The escort consisted of 51 P-51s from the 55 FG, 40 from the 78 FG, 47 from the 339 FG, 40 from the 353 FG, and 53 from the 357 FG.*

[24] *IV/JG 301 came into existence in the autumn of 1944 from III/KG 'Hindenburg' (that had flown He 177s before) and that was why it retained the original combat name, rather than 'Wilde Sau' to which it never belonged.*

P-51D 44-71228 "Big Beautiful Doll", 78 FG, personal aircraft of Col. John D. Landers.
P. Randall via R. Abbey

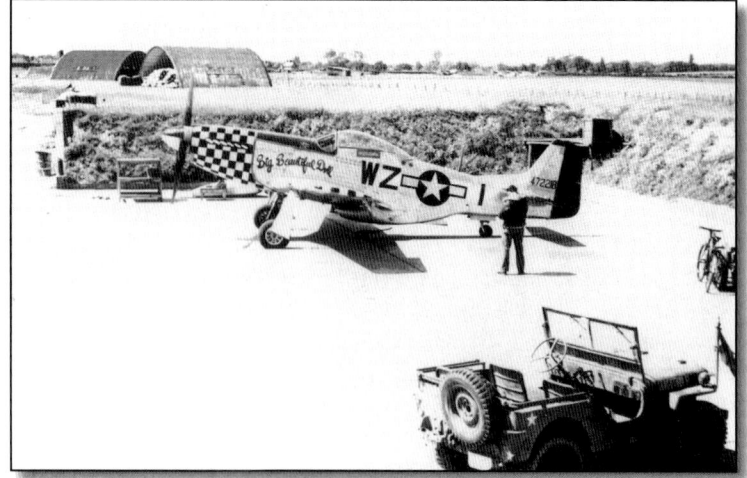

probably confused by the damaged and burning machines.

Two pilots of the 364 FS 357 FG finished off the Bf 109G-10 (W. Nr.491200) 'yellow 7' over Burg. The first of these, Capt. Robert G. Schimanski, reported: *'I was leading the blue flight, when enemy fighters were reported east of Magdeburg. Down below me I saw an explosion, so I headed there with my section. At an altitude of about 10,000 feet (3,000 m) I recognized one Me 109. I jettisoned my drop tanks and attacked. The lone 109 followed four P-51s from the 339 FG. After about five minutes of tough combat one of the 339 FG pilots was hit perfectly several times. The 109 spun out of combat and the 339 aircraft did not follow. I kept track of the enemy aircraft.*

Under the clouds the German attacked first and combat began again. After another five minutes of head-on attacks I was joined by Lt Karger. We started to fire at him together, and this proved effective. Lt Karger hit the German near the cockpit and he attempted to escape downwards. I followed him and fired at him until he crashed on the ground.

1/Lt Dale E. Karger reported: *'The Me 109 continued to spin, so I pulled the controls lightly, until I entered a shallow dive. This was enough to fire one burst precisely into the cockpit. Then I saw Capt. Schimanski who hung behind the tail of my German, fired again and left, so that I could act again. When I fired for the first time, I must have hit the pilot, because his machine started to fall flatly and hit the ground. The wings broke away from the fuselage and fire burst out. Then the wreckage was strafed by Capt. Schimanski, and I followed him to take photos with the camera gun. I claim one Me 109 destroyed in co-operation with Capt. Schimanski.*

The machine had a white whirl on the black propeller cone, and a red band with two yellow ones on the fuselage. There was a large yellow 7 on the fuselage aft of the cockpit'.

The victors of the German pilot are thus known, but varying identities of the victim are quoted in various sources. According to the identification bands the machine came from JG 301[25]. According to the data of W. Girbig, this pointed to Herald Ruh who lost his life over Stresow. On the other hand, German archival materials link the machine, according to its Werk

[25] *When identifying the machine according to the Reich Defence bands, the Bf 109 can be considered part of JG 301. Even if JG 301 usually used only two bands: yellow and red, there are known cases where triple bands were used, or the sequence of colours was reversed.*

Nummer, to IV/JG 300. On 2 March this was apparently flown by Fhr. Arno Schmidt[26] who was killed over Burg. In the area of the 357 FG's combat with enemy fighters more machines from IV/JG 300 crashed, but not a single one from IV/JG 301. This fought further to the north of the 339 and 78 FG. It is not impossible, however, that in this giant melee, individual units got mixed.

The case of III/JG 301 was interesting. Its pilots took off from Sachau in a force of 10-12 Fw 190A-8 and A-9, and 10 Ta 152H-0 and H-1 machines. Upon take-off they headed south, towards Harz. According to the ground controller, they were going to encounter another group of German fighters there. The Focke Wulf Fw 190As formed a combat formation, and the Ta 152s provided cover to them at an altitude of 8,000 m. Another group of German fighters appeared in the distance. When they got closer, they did not join the III/JG 301 machines, but mistook these for the enemy and attacked the Ta 152s. Uffz. Blum was bounced by one of the first, but thanks to the excellent flying characteristics and manoeuvrability of the Ta 152 he evaded the attack unharmed. It took no uncertain terms from Oblt. Stahl, the Ta 152 group leader, to make the situation clear and quiet. However, after this incident the formation broke, and the Ta 152 pilots were so furious and confused that they returned to base immediately.

The rest of III/JG 301 engaged the escort fighters without losses. One of the 9 Staffel pilots, Lt. August-Wilhelm Hagedorn, even managed to shoot down a B-17 over Magdeburg.

III/JG 300 lost five machines and three pilots in combat. These included Hptm. Peter Jenne, commander of III Gruppe, recently awarded his Knight's Cross. His Messerschmitt G-10 'blue 1' crashed at Niemegen. Jenne was born on 5 May 1920 at Wittenburg/Sachsen. In 1943 he had been a 'Zerstörer' pilot in I/ZG 26 in Reich Defence, against American bombers. Later, as the Staffelkapitän of 12/JG 300 he performed many attacks against ground targets. He had also enjoyed success against the 'heavies', for example on 17 December 1944, when he downed two Liberators in his G-10. When decorated with the Knight's Cross, on 2 February 1945, he already had 17 aerial victories to his credit, including 12 four-engined bombers, plus 12 tanks, 10 self-propelled guns and 8 rocket launchers destroyed on the ground.

But the Americans also suffered losses. Lt Patrick Mallione from the 357 FG was hit during a dog fight with pilots from JG 300. His P-51D was last seen 40 km north of Leipzig. 1/Lt Glenwood A. Zarnke of the 363 FS 357 FG reported: *'On March 2, 1945, on a combat mission I was flying in #3 position in Cement Yellow flight. Capt. Robert Moore was flying #1 position. The last time I saw Lt Mallione was when he sighted an Me109 coming in from 11 o'clock. Capt. Moore dropped his tanks as I dropped mine and I looked back and saw Mallione behind me. He had not dropped his tanks as yet, but I presumed he did and followed us. Both Capt. Moore and I went into compressibility in the dive after the Me109. When we recovered Lt Mallione was not to be seen. We both called to him on the R/T but received no answer. These events took place at 10.20 hours at a point 10 miles south of Wittenberg.'*

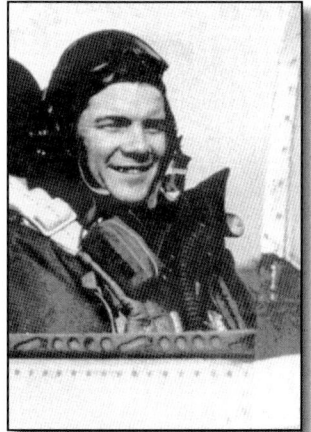

1/Lt. Dale E. Karger, 357 FG. 357 FG Assn.

[26] The matter is not clarified even by the official German war grave care organisation (Volksbund Deutsche Kriegsgräberfürsorge e.V.). Its data base does not include Arno Schmidt under 2 March, but it mentions Harald Ruh born on 15 March 1925, killed on 2 March 1945. He is buried at the Kriegsgräberstätte in Burg (row 3, grave 5).

An Ordinary Day in 1945

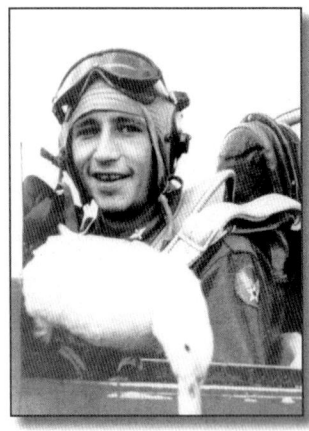

Capt. Robert G. Schimansky, 357 FG, one of the two US pilots, who determined the fate of German pilot Harald Ruh.

357 FG Assn.

[27] RLM- Ic Reich Tagesmel-dung for 2 March 1945 states that 198 aircraft were airborne against enemy heavy bombers over central Germany, claiming 24 victories. Eight of these should be due to JG 301 pilots. But we know that they claimed only two bombers, so we may expect huge overclaiming in this report.

[28] He is buried at Lorraine American Cemetery, St. Avold, France (Plot A, Row 15, Gr. 61).

One I/JG 300 pilot claimed a Mustang shot down north of Wittenberg. This was the sole victory of the Germans over American fighters. However, not all claims have survived or are available in the archives. Therefore it is not impossible that there may have been more German claims[27].

Capt. Alva C. Murphy from the 364 FS was another 357 FG pilot lost in the combat. South of Magdeburg he and his wingman 1/Lt H. Wesling entered combat with Bf 109s. Wesling gave the following account in the MACR: *'I was flying greenhouse red two, wingman to Capt. Murphy. Southeast of Magdeburg we spotted a Me 109 in the clouds at approximately 5000 feet. We were at approx. 6000 feet and dove down and closed on the Me 109 to within 300 yards. Capt. Murphy started firing at about 40 to 50 degree deflection and I observed hits around the wings and cockpit. The Me 109 flipped over and went straight in; no chute.*

About five minutes later we saw another Me 109 below the clouds at approx. 3000 feet. We dove on this Me 109 and began turning with the e/a. After about two turns Captain Murphy got strikes on the 109 and it burst into flames and crashed.

After a few minutes we spotted an airfield and Capt. Murphy and I went down. Capt. Murphy was hit by Flak in his coolant. We pulled up to about 3,000 feet and after a few minutes his engine quit. He rolled over and bailed out approximately 30 miles southeast of Magdeburg. His chute did open, but I did not follow him down.'

The P-51D 44-63765 crashed near Gröbzig, killing the pilot. Murphy was posthumously promoted to Major. He is buried in the Luxembourg American Cemetery (plot G, row 7, grave 23). His decorations included Air Medal with 11 Gold Stars, and Purple Heart. He had 6 victories to his credit.

The fate of Capt. Murphy was shared by 1/Lt Mathew Crawford from the 363 FS. His P-51D 44-15161 'Joyce', damaged by Flak, crashed near Creuzburg in Germany[28], killing the pilot.

1/Lt R.R. LePore in the P-51 D 44-14555 'Pretty Pat' was the last Flak victim from the 357 FG. He managed to bale out of the damaged aircraft and he was taken prisoner.

The 339 FG also encountered some 35 German Bf 109 and Fw 190 fighters, probably of IV/JG 301, II, III and IV/JG 300. For this unit this was the first engagement with the enemy in the new year, and it completely compensated for the long period of combat 'abstinence'. Its pilots claimed 14-2-8 air victories and 11-0-3 enemy machines destroyed on the ground.

1/Lt Lawrence Poutre from the 503 FS claimed 2 Bf 109s and one Fw 190 destroyed.

'I was leading Beefsteak Black Flight, in Red Section, when we sighted two gaggles of enemy aircraft below us. Red and White flights attacked the lower gaggle, made up of Fw 190s (probably II/JG 300, author's note), while I took my flight down on their top cover of Me 109s (most probably III/JG 300, author's note).

I closed to very short range on the last man in the formation, fired a short burst from 20 degrees deflection, and the 109 exploded in a sheet of flame.

I pulled up and attacked a 190 and, after a little maneuvering, got into position to fire. I gave him a short burst from very short range and saw strikes on his wing root and canopy. At this point my wingman, Lt Sams overshot me in a turn and I called him to break because he had a 109 on his tail. Lt Sams then attacked the 190 I´d been firing at but did no shooting because the enemy aircraft was on fire and going down out of control.

As the Me 109 chasing Lt Sams passed me I got into position and fired a slight deflection burst. The enemy aircraft caught fire and the pilot jettisoned his canopy and bailed out.'

Also Capt. James R. Starnes from the 505 FS 339 FG had a successful fight:

'I was leading Upper Blue Section on a Ramrod to Ruhland. On penetration just east of Magdeburg, Beefsteak called in bandits approaching from low and to the right of our first box of bombers. I took my flight into the dogfight and dropped tanks after identifying the bandits as Me 109s. The enemy I claim as destroyed was on the tail of a P-51 from the 78 FG from Duxford. We went into a tight Luftberry to the left and I do not think that the 109 was able to draw enough lead to fire at the P-51. My first burst fell a bit short and, as I corrected with a tighter turn, several strikes appeared on the left wing and fuselage. He reefed it in harder and broke for the clouds.

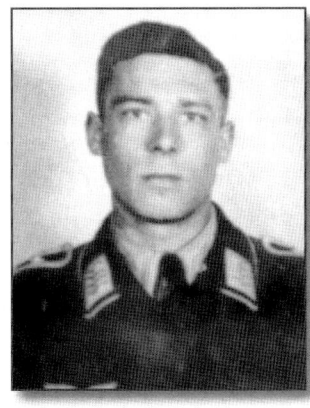

Above:
Hptm. Peter Jenne died in the combat with US fighters. He received the Ritterkreuz one month before his last action, on 2nd February

So I tucked in underneath him and waited for another crack as the enemy aircraft pulled wing tip streamers at 450 m.p.h. in the pull-out under the cloud deck. Apparently, he figured that I had been shaken as he flew straight for a few seconds. I fired another burst at 300 yards and hit his left radiator intake. He attempted skidding and slipping tactics but I put a long burst into his engine and port fuselage from five degree deflection. The engine burst into flames and then the whole thing caught fire. Pieces flew off as the aircraft did a violent snap roll to the left and went into a normal spin at 2,000 feet. The pilot did not bail out but I believe that canopy was jettisoned. This 109 had a fixed tail wheel but there were no visible braces on the tail. There was a vertical red band around a fuselage.'
Based on the markings observation, this Bf 109 belonged to III or IV/JG 300.

Below:
Lt. August - Wilhelm Hagedorn from 9./JG 301, who claimed a B-17 on March 2, 1945.
via W. Reschke

'Other members of my Flight followed me and attacked Me109s. Lt Jay Marts claimed two enemy aircraft shot down in head to head attacks. Lt John Withers and Lt Harry Ziegler shared the fourth Me109 claimed by the pilots of my Flight that day.'

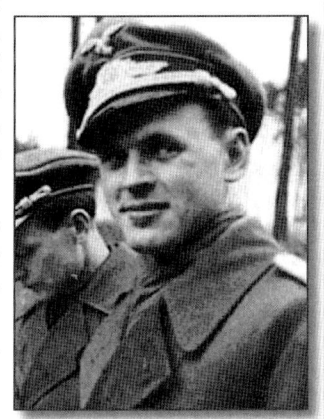

Also the 353 FG took part in the encounter with Fw190s, most probably from II/JG 300 and JGr. 10, and with Messerschmitts from IV/JG 300. Several kilometres south-east of Magdeburg, near Wittenburg, its pilots claimed seven Bf 109s and ten Fw 190s destroyed. Lt Col. William B. Bailey, the CO 353 FG, claimed two Fw 190s south of Wittenburg, most probably from II Gruppe JG 300.

The Sturmgruppe of Waldemar 'Waldi' Radener (II/JG 300), after their successful attack against the bombers in which its pilots claimed five B-17s shot down in the Torgau area, had to join the combat with fighters and lost six machines and four pilots. Ofw. Richard Löfgen, victor in 12 combats, was shot down in his 'green 2' not far from Groß Treben, north of Torgau. Two more pilots from 5/JG 300, Fh. Siegfried Felske and Uffz. Karl Werner (born on 10 March 1923 at Immelborn) also lost their lives in that area. Fh. Felske is buried at Anneburg, while Uffz. Werner has no known grave and he is considered missing.

An Ordinary Day in 1945

Right: F/O Patrick J. Mallione, 357 FG, 363 FS.
Below: Capt. Alva C. Murphy, 357 FG. 364 FS.
both via M. Olmsted

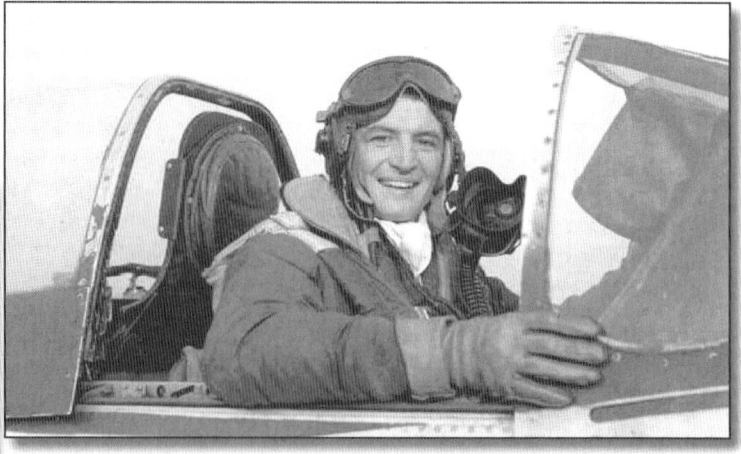

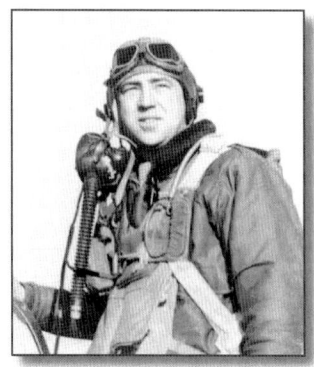

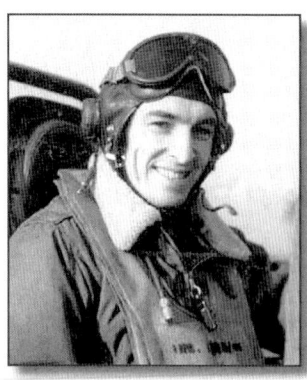

Above: 1/Lt. Mathew Crawford, 357 FG, 363 FS.
Below: 1/Lt. Rocco R. LePore, 357 FG, 364 FS.
both via M. Olmsted

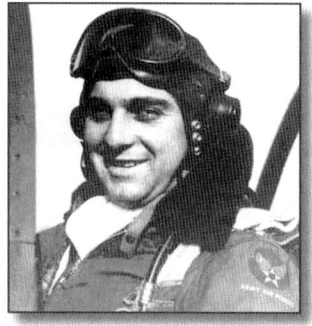

Also JGr. 10 lost four Fw 190A-8s in this area and two pilots: Ofw. Hermann Brennicke in 'black 3' and Ofw. Rudolf Schimmelpfenig in 'black 4' were both killed.

According to the German historian Werner Girbig, JG 300, JG 301 and JGr. 10, all reporting to IX Fligerkorps, lost a total of 53 machines in the combats, achieving 15 victories. Unfortunately, I was not able to establish a detailed list of claims due to incomplete archives. So far six victories of JG 300 and two claims by JG 301 pilots are known.

On the other hand, American pilots from the Task Force II escort claimed 54-3-16 enemy machines destroyed in the air and 36-0-24 on the ground. They lost 13 machines with pilots killed or captured. Three more machines returned damaged.

The enemy machines destroyed on the ground fell prey to two groups: 339 FG and 357 FG which, having chased away the Germans, left the bombers and headed down. Pilots of the 339 FG claimed 11-0-4 and those from the 357 FG 33-0-20 enemy aircraft destroyed on the ground.

Pilots of the 505 FS 339 FG attacked a Luftwaffe aerodrome with dispersed aircraft. Their claims included 11 Do 217s destroyed and 2 Do 217s damaged. Lt Briggs, Lt Burch and Lt Howard destroyed three Do 217s each, two Do217s were claimed destroyed on the ground by Lt Conner, and two damaged by Lt Biggs. Capt. Starnes also claimed a Mistel, composed of a Ju 88 and an Fw 190, as damaged on the ground. *'...After shooting down the Me 109 I was under the clouds at an altitude of about 1,500 feet. I then saw a grass airfield with a lot of Mistels there, hidden under trees and covered with branches. I attacked one of these and damaged it. It did not catch fire, though. I had little ammunition and fuel, so I concentrated on noting the precise location of the airfield. Upon return to Fowlmere I pointed that out and the next day we returned. I destroyed one Mistel. But after the previous experience the Germans were prepared and ground fire shot down two our machines'.*

The claims for the Do 217s must have been a case of misidentification, as the Luftwaffe recorded no loss of the type that day. The aerodrome attacked by Mustangs from the 339 FG was probably Alten-Grabow, situated near Möckern. At the time this was the base of II/KG 200. Its inventory included

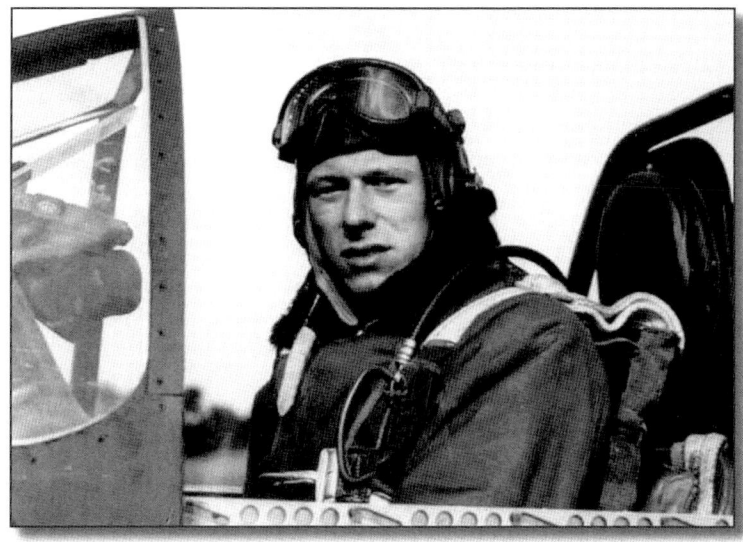

Left: 1/Lt. Raymond M. Bank, 357 FG, 364 FS

via M. Olmsted

An Ordinary Day in 1945

Fw 190s and Ju 88s in Mistel combinations. Following the attack of American fighters on 2 March 1945 it lost several machines. Five were 100% destroyed, while eight more aircraft, Fw 190s or Ju 88s, were 10-15% damaged (see loss listings). The aerodrome had good defence, and its AA fire claimed one 339 FG machine. Its pilot, 1/Lt Harry F. Howard (O-710115) was forced to spend some time in Germany (POW).

'On 2 March 1945 Bert Conner was leading the upper Green Flight escorting B-17s during the attack on Berlin (sic). Kenneth Biggs was flying as wingman to Bert. I was an element leader, with Hal Burch as my wingman. Not far from the target we spotted several Me 109s. We left the escort and chased the Germans in vain, as they hid in clouds. Our flight started to look for targets of opportunity under the clouds. We located a motorway area about 40 miles (65 km) east of Magdeburg. German aircraft were collected there. They were all perfectly camouflaged under trees. We found them thanks to ruts left by vehicle wheels towards the trees. Bert checked the area for AA weapons. As we met no opposition, we started to attack the dispersed machines by individual elements. After a few attacks we ran out of ammunition. Then Bert said that he was hit and that he turned home. I commenced the last attack. I turned back and made sure my tail was clean. My next recollection was when I woke up several days later in a German hospital for prisoners. Bert Conner was lying in the bed next to me. I could not recall what happened, so I wanted to get up and fly back to England'.

What Howard omitted, is added by the account of Hal Burch, included in the Missing Air Crew Report:

'On the March 2, 1945 I was flying number four position on Lt H. F. Howard's wing. We had come down on the deck in search of reported enemy aircraft when Lt Biggs spotted some enemy aircraft hidden in a wood and broke off to strafe them. Lt Howard followed with myself bringing up the rear. We established a gunnery pattern making left hand passes. Lt Howard and myself on one end of the woods, Lt Conner and Lt

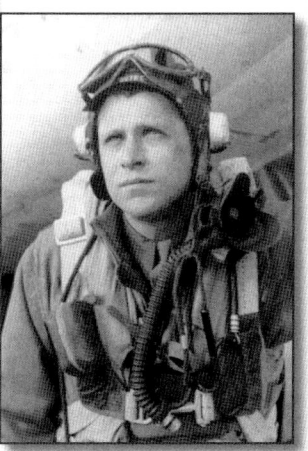

1/Lt Lawrence Poutre, 339 FG, 503 FS.

via 339 FG Assn.

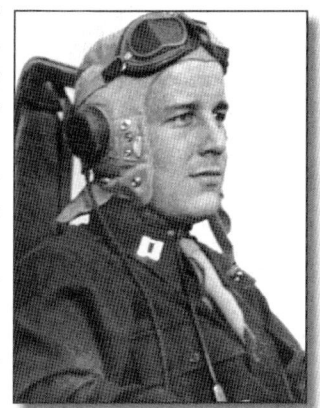

Capt. James R. Starnes, 339 FG, 505 FS.

via 339 FG Assn.

An Ordinary Day in 1945

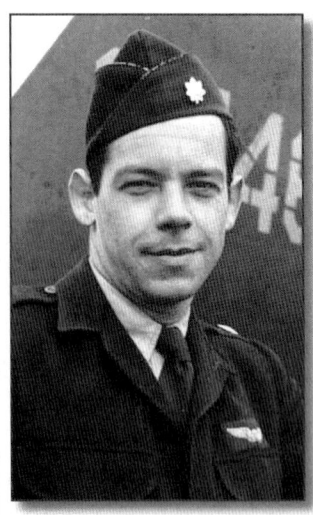

Above:
Lt. Col. William Bradford Bailey, 353 FG, 352 FS, who shot down two Fw 190s on March 2.
via 353 FG Assn.

Below:
Lt. Waldemar Radener, Gruppenkommandeur II/JG 300. In February 1943 came to II/ JG 26 as young Leutenant. Moved to II/JG 300 having been Gruppenkommandeur II/JG 26. Ten day after the March 2 action was awarded by Ritterkreutz. During WWII claimed 36 victories - all in the west (including 16 four-engined bombers).
via D. Caldwell

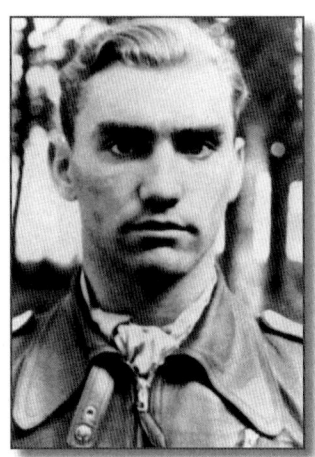

Biggs on the other end firing at enemy aircraft. We had made about five passes when Lt Biggs and Lt Conner left the pattern. I had exhausted my ammunition then but evidently Lt Howard had not as he stayed low and in the pattern went up for another pass. I followed him around, still behind him and a little higher as I did not intend to make a pass, as I was turning off the base leg onto the approach to the targets. I saw Lt Howard pull up just above the aircraft he had been firing on and crash into the trees. I flew over the spot and could see the wreckage strew through the trees. There was no fire, I circled the spot about five minutes but could see no movement or fire. I do not believe Lt Howard could have escaped. The time was approximately 11.30 hours and in the vicinity of Möckern. Lt Howard was flying a P-51D-10 44-14622.'

The machine had previously been used by Jim Robinson, who returned to the USA on 23 February. The aircraft then had no 'owner' and on 2 March 1945 'Little One II' left the ground for the last time.

'The Flak that got me', continued Lt Howard, 'hit my left leg. The blow had probably thrown me out of the cockpit and I landed among trees on a telephone line that miraculously slowed down my flight from 300 mph (500 km/h) to zero without major injuries. That just was not my day to die.

Together with Bert Conner we remained at the Stalag XI-A hospital until we were liberated by the US Army in May 1945. Then we were moved to the 10th Evacuation Hospital at Magdeburg. On VE Day we were taken to Paris. At the end of 1946 I got my Purple Heart and promotion to Capt.'

As mentioned above, also Capt. Bert Conner ended up in the hospital:

'The flight continued without major incidents until a place somewhere east of Magdeburg, where we attacked several Me 109s. They attacked the red section and approached us in combat formation. But they headed into clouds, where they disappeared. I thought we would play it cool and fly around the clouds until some of them appeared. We flew around for a while, but then I cancelled the action and with the flight we tracked the ruts left by vehicles from the motorway to the woods where they disappeared. To our surprise we found a big number of aircraft hidden under trees. I called the flight and warned them to watch out until I checked the area for AA weapons. After the search was negative, we started to destroy the dispersed aircraft.

I was coming in for the last attack. When I got over the trees the world exploded. I wondered why I could not move my rudder to the left. I looked down and realised that my left leg was bent under the seat. I could not pull it out. I only pulled it out using my hands. I turned for home. I looked at the compass, took heading west, moved the throttle fully open. Then I tried to stop my bleeding. For a moment I felt terrible pain and I fainted for a short while. When I becamet conscious again, the aircraft flew very slow and thick smoke drew behind me. I was at an altitude of about 500 feet (150 m), so I could not even think of baling out until I got higher. I then spotted a glade in the wood ahead of me. In fact this was a German Luftwaffe landing ground. I headed for the right side of the runway. I forced-landed on the grass. When my 'Lone Star Lady' came to a halt I unfastened my harness. The aircraft was not on fire, so I did not hurry. I injected myself a dose of morphine into my leg. Then I realised somebody was standing above me. The German soldier saw my wounds but did nothing until an ambulance came. They pulled me out of the aircraft, placed me on stretchers, and took me to the main building. The dressed my wounds provisionally. Later after lunch they took me in a car, perhaps of 1920, to Stalag XI-A at Altengrabow. We arrived there by dark. Several men started to interrogate me then. They spoke very good English. In the morning I was moved to a room where about ten other men lay. I looked around and saw Lt Howard lying next to me.'

Mustangs of the 357 FG also found a suitable target on the ground and were able to bring valuable claims back home. Several flights of the 357 FG got low over the grass surface of the aerodrome located at rd9290-9897 co-ordinates[29], which housed over 200 enemy machines of all types, dispersed under trees in the wood to the east, west and north of the airfield. American pilots destroyed 15 and damaged 16 machines. The pilots said that this must have been a storage ground for Luftwaffe machines. They saw Fw 190s, He 111s, Ju 88s dispersed all over the woods. The aircraft were partly camouflaged, looked new, mostly still in natural metal. Piles of fuselage and wing components were located on the outskirts.

The aerodrome was poorly defended from the ground. Only one gun started to fire, but it was effective. Two machines were damaged and one was missing from the action, probably due to a direct hit.

One unit of the 357 FG attacked the aerodrome at Kamenz (sa4418 co-ordinates), destroying ten enemy aircraft and damaging four, including a number of Mistels. AA defences of the aerodrome were silent throughout the attack.

After the action American pilots from the 357 FG claimed the following targets destroyed on the ground: 19-0-17 T/E, 6-0-3 S/E[30] including 6-0-2 Mistels at the Grabow/Zietlow aerodrome[31], 3-0-0 locomotives and 5-0-0 military vehicles destroyed on the motorway at rz4303 co-ordinates (now A9 motorway in Germany).

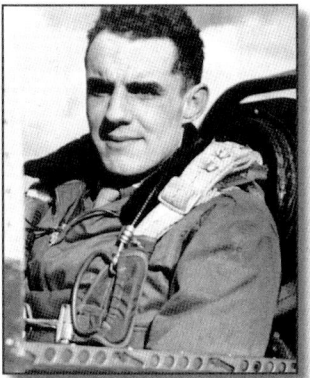

Above:
1/Lt. Harry F. Howard, 339 FG, 505 FS.

via 339 FG Assn.

[29] *According to co-ordinates this was an airfield located between Buhlendorf and Wahl, south of Möckern.*

[30] *T/E – twin-engined (aircraft), S/E – single-engined.*

[31] *Probably the 357 FG pilots attacked the base of II/KG 200 together with the 339 FG. This explains the presence of unidentified American fighters attacking the aerodrome at Grabow, as shown in the sketch by Lt Biggs.*

Claims of 357 FG pilots for targets destroyed on the ground

Claim	Status	Pilot	FS	Note
4 He111	destroyed	Lt Robinson	362	
2 He111	destroyed	Lt Beecraft	362	
2 He111	destroyed	Lt Beecraft	362	part of a Mistel
2 Fw190	destroyed	Lt Beecraft	362	part of a Mistel
1 He111	damaged	Lt Beecraft	362	
1 He111	damaged	Lt Robinson	362	

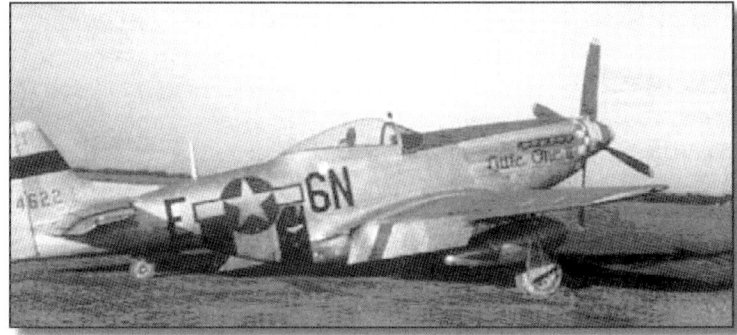

Left:
Harry Howard's plane P-51D 44-14622 "Little One II", 339 FG, still wearing D-Day stripes. Photo is dated to late 1944.

via 339 FG Assn.

An Ordinary Day in 1945

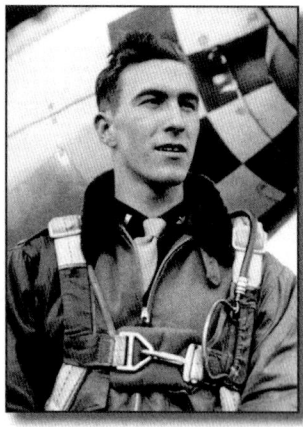

*Lt. Halard Burch of 339 FG.
via 339 FG Assn.*

1 He111	damaged	Lt Robinson	362	part of a Mistel
1 Fw190	damaged	Lt Robinson	362	part of a Mistel
4 He111	destroyed	Lt Zettler	364	
2 He111	destroyed	Lt Williams	364	
1 He111	destroyed	Lt Hohes	364	
2 He111	destroyed	Capt. Schimanski	364	part of a Mistel
2 He111	destroyed	Lt Karger	364	part of a Mistel
2 Fw190	destroyed	Capt. Schimanski	364	part of a Mistel
2 Fw190	destroyed	Lt Karger	364	part of a Mistel
8 He111	damaged	Lt Williams	364	
3 Ju88	damaged	Lt Karger	364	
1 Ju188	damaged	Lt Karger	364	
1 He111	damaged	Lt Wesling	364	
1 He111	damaged	Lt Williams	364	part of a Mistel
1 Fw190	damaged	Lt Williams	364	part of a Mistel
1 Fw190	damaged	Lt Karger	364	

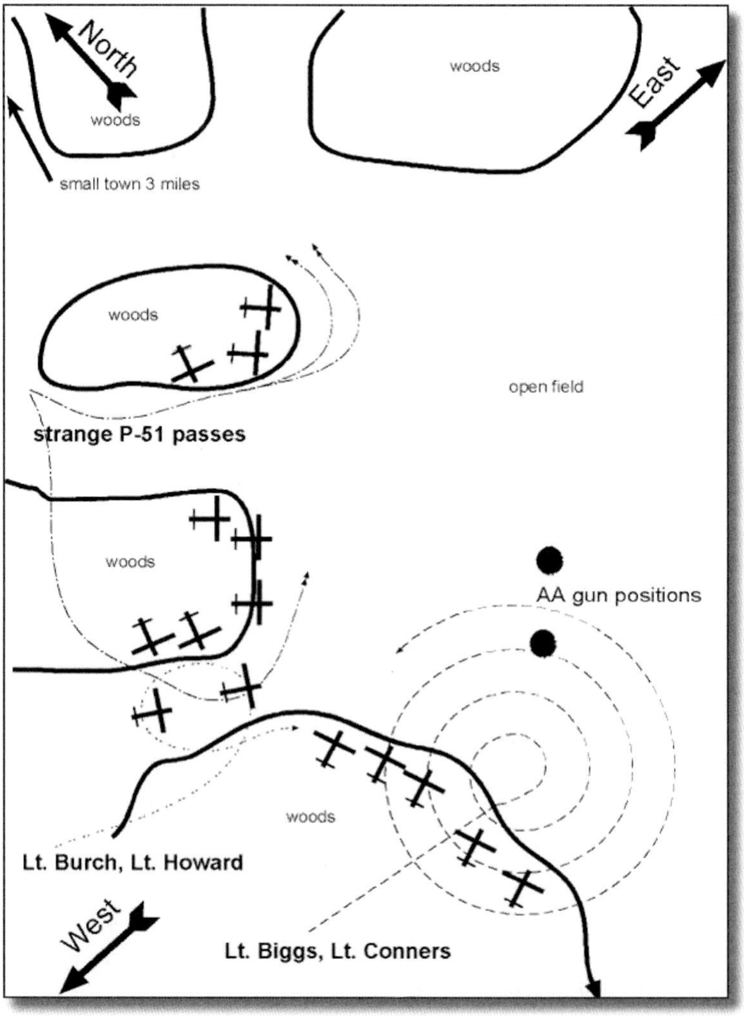

*Right:
Drawing by Lt Biggs from the 339 FG, depicting the strafing attack at the aerodrome on 2 March 1945*

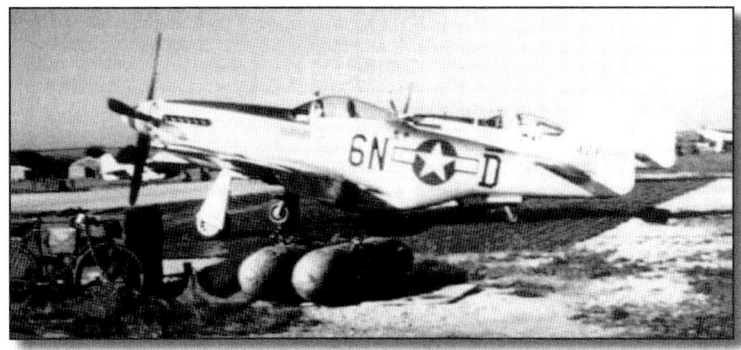

Left:
Plane of Lt. Harald W. Burch. This P-51D 44-72098 (6N-D) belonged to 505 FS, 339 FG.
via 339 FG Assn.

In concluding it is worth adding an interesting piece of information about claims filed by bomber gunners. They claimed a total of 31 German fighters. The most, 11 shot down, were claimed by upper turret gunners, while 10 were claimed by tail gunners. This would mean much higher losses on the German side than were really inflicted. There is nothing unusual about gunners claiming so many more kills than could have taken place. After a gunner fired his bursts at a fast flying enemy fighter, the latter would disappear from his sight and the gunner was unable to track its further fate. Moreover, if a German pilot accelerated or slowed down, and his machine's engine produced darker exhaust gases, the gunner believed he had hit the enemy and claimed its destruction. One has to taken yet another aspect into account. Several gunners were likely to aim at one and take the same German machine, so such an alleged kill may have been claimed by several men.

Task Force III

321 B-24 Liberators of the 2nd Air Division took off from their bases in south-east England at 06.25-07.59. They crossed the Channel and the Dutch coast, and headed towards the Dummer lake (Dummer See) north of Brunswick. Fighter escort was provided by a mixed formation of 195 Mustangs and Thunderbolts. The exact numbers were as follows: 46 P-51s from the 4 FG, 22 P-47s from the 56 FG, 29 Mustangs from the 355 FG, 50 P-51s from the 361 FG, and 48 P-51s from the 479 FG. Task Force III was also accompanied by nine P-51s from the 862 BS that flew a weather reconnaissance mission. Fighter escorts patrolled ahead of the bomber formation over the Zuider Zee area and the Dutch-German border.

Due to strong winds, Task Force III was several minutes behind the scheduled time of arrival over the target. Over Magdeburg the bomber crews encountered sky with 8/10 cloud cover.

The primary target, the synthetic oil plant Braunkohle-Benzin at Magdeburg/Rothensee, was bombed by 45 Liberators of parts of the 491 FG and 392 BG, and of the entire 446 BG. Between 03.15-04.30 hours 21 crews of the 392 BG were selected and after morning procedures they took off at 07.00 on a mission They dropped their bomb load on the target from an altitude of 22,000-24,200 feet (6,700-7,400 m) at 10.37-10.41. The north-east and south-east part of the target area was hit. Thick black smoke rose from the buildings that were hit. Photos taken the following day proved that the attack was precise and most of the target was heavily damaged or destroyed.

Due to bad cloud cover over the primary target the 446 BG decided to attack the secondary target. But en route the CO located a gap in clouds which allowed the crews 446 BG to carry out their primary duty and they dropped their bombs over the primary target, inline astern.

The secondary target, the marshalling yard at Magdeburg/Buckau was attacked by most machines of Task Force III. A total of 227 B-24s dropped their bombs using the H2X system from an altitude of 21,400-24,000 feet (6,500-7,300 m) between 10.34 and 10.46. The station buildings and neighbouring areas were destroyed. Also hit was the Fried Krupp Werke factory, situated not far from the station. Virtually all buildings and equipment in the target area were hit.

Bombers of Task Force III also attacked some targets of opportunity. A complete combat formation of the 466 BG attacked a refinery in the town of Schonebeck. At 10.46 bombs from 21 aircraft fell from 22,500-23,000 feet (6,900-7,000 m) and exploded on the ground. This attack lasted three and a half minutes.

Task Force III bombers dropped a total of 456 tonnes of bombs on their targets. Of this 108 tonnes was dropped by 45 aircraft on the primary targets, 573 tonnes of bombs from 227 aircraft on the secondary targets, and 21 aircraft dropped 75 tonnes of bombs on targets of opportunity.

The Task Force III fighter escort which, as mentioned before, consisted of four Mustangs groups and one Thunderbolt group, was supposed to defend its bombers as best it could. For this reason one section of Mustangs of one group detached and flew far ahead to the Berlin area, in order to attack the Germans already on the way in and to break their formations. But not a single Luftwaffe fighter waited for the approaching bombers over Magdeburg or the neighbouring area. Task Force III bombers dropped their bombs and headed for home. They were the first to cross the English coast, which serves as a proof that they were not slowed down by enemy activity. Only one group was behind its schedule by some 10-35 minutes. This was due to a navigation error. The crews corrected this in time and returned safely home. The fighters that escorted the Liberators spotted one Fw 190 attacking a marauding bomber south-east of Magdeburg and easily chased it away to a safe distance.

Despite the problem-free mission, escort pilots from the 355 FG claimed 5-2-0 victories. Between 10.20 and 10.45 in the area of Dummer Lake up to north-east Koblenz, just one pilot of the 358 FS 355 FG, 1/Lt

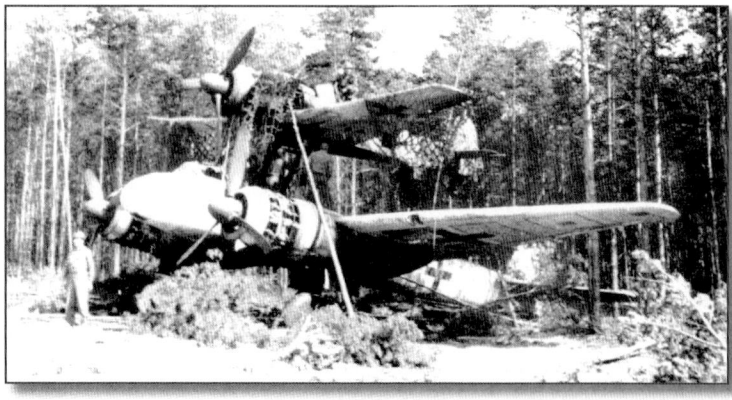

Damaged Mistel Fw 190/Ju 88 partially hidden under the trees on the abandoned field.

Roscoe R. Allen, claimed five Bf 109s destroyed. In his report he wrote:

'Following a failure of the oxygen system I abandoned the escort sortie and turned back home. About 10.20 in the Dummer Lake area I saw 15 Me 109s with bombs attached[32]. They had yellow-red markings and dragon motifs[33]. From an altitude of about 6,000 feet (2,000 m) I attacked the upper of the two groups. I carried out the attack from the sun, thus unseen. After the successful attack I fired again and with my burst I hit another Me 109 which started to smoke. The pilot baled out. The third Me 109 turned upside down after having taken a few hits. The lower group broke apart. I attacked five machines that remained relatively together. The pilot of the fourth machine that I damaged baled out.'

Lt Allen's final confirmed victim headed for clouds. After a long burst a flame appeared on the Bf 109. The pilot fired another burst on yet another Bf 109 which then disappeared in clouds. Then a German fighter appeared behind him, and a classic dogfight commenced in which both machines were hit. Lt Allen last saw the Bf 109 at an altitude of some 15 m over the ground and with a damaged engine. He claimed the last two as probably destroyed.

During the raid, Task Force III lost three bombers. Liberator B-24 J 42-51302 from the 576 BS 392 BG was lost en route to the target. It was hit by an unfortunate burst from a neighbouring bomber as machine guns were tested. Information about the circumstances of the event was provided in the MACR by two S/Sgts: Joseph G. Coffman and Robert E. Ruigh: 'Tracers were seen going into A/C 42-51302. Fire appeared in the cockpit and the plane peeled off seeming to be under control. Went down in a slow wide circle into the clouds trailing smoke. A total of five (5) chutes were seen.' The blame for the accident was placed on the rear gunner of 42-29476 which flew as the leader of the top section.

German materials say that the bomber crashed at 12.00 some 9 km north-east of Lubbicke, south-east of Osnabrück near Detmold. Five crew members were taken prisoner, and five burnt bodies were recovered from the wreckage. Those dead crew members were buried in the local cemetery, and after the end of the war their remains were taken to the cemetery at Liege. Capt. Blakeley was posthumously awarded the Purple Heart.

In the B-24 J 44-40436 'Nancy' from the 578 BS 392 BG, flown by 2/Lt Downs, waist gunner Sgt E.W. Cinquina was killed by a direct Flak hit.

Two other lost machines were from the 466 BG and 467 BG. The B-24 J 42-51273 from the 785 BS 466 BG, flown by 2/Lt H.W.Greiner, was officially declared missing. According to eyewitnesses the machine was hit by Fw190 fire somewhere over Dummer See. Nine parachutes were seen, but the co-pilot Edmund B. Knoll, navigator Andrew L. Swarz, waist gunner Robert E. Shaddy and tail gunner Ernest H. Ratliff never returned home. They were killed in action. Nothing more precise is known about the other crew members, only that they become Prisoners of War. This was their second mission. The machine crashed near Tenneheide.

The last Liberator, B-24H-25-DT 42-51171 'Eli Sworf Jr' from the 790 BS 467 BG lost one engine over the target. Another engine stopped working after an attack by German fighters. The machine left formation and was hit by Flak. It started to burn. Sgt Edward N. Gibbs described the events:

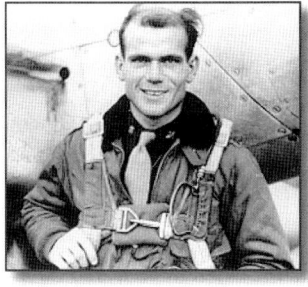

Lt. Kenneth Biggs, eye witness of Lt. Howard's terrible crash and miraculous survival.

via 339 FG Assn.

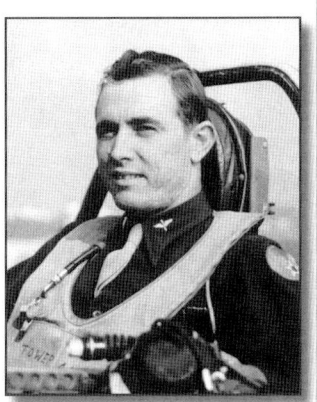

Capt. Bert Conner, member of 339 Fighter Group.

via 339 FG Assn.

[32] *Probably drop tanks.*

[33] *The markings suggest that it was almost certainly IV/JG 301 flying Bf109s. Pilots of the group were young, mostly without any combat experience, which explains why their behaviour in combat against Lt Allen allowed the US pilot to claim five victories.*

An Ordinary Day in 1945

'We left England about 05.15 and headed for Magdeburg. About 05.30 we arrived over enemy territory, the line was easy to recognise by the small puffs of black smoke from AA fire everywhere around our aircraft. This lasted for a few seconds, followed by six and half hours of silence.

Approximately at 12.00 our machine was hit in the left inboard engine. Due to this we were not able to stay in formation, so we headed for the nearest Allied territory. It all took about 5 minutes. We were then about 1,000 feet over the ground and Flak started to fire at us madly. We all started to pray. And then it happened. A direct hit exploded no further than two feet right of the rear gunner and myself. After a few seconds I got conscious enough to realise I was falling in the air. I quickly reached for the ripcord, but it was not there. I looked up and saw my parachute was open. I fell on the ground and tried to get out of my parachute. Both my legs were broken, so I unfastened my parachute harness lying down.

Soon afterwards a group of Germans came. They had knives and firearms in their hands. Soon they left, leaving one man on guard'.

The wounded airman was then taken by the Germans to the hospital at Leeuwarden in the Netherlands, where he remained until 15 April 1945, when he was liberated by the Canadian 3rd Army. Four members of the crew of 2/Lt Alvah D. Reid baled out. One of the parachutes failed to open and the airman was killed. The other six men died in the machine that crashed at Dorstend near Essen.

In this combat 53 bombers were damaged, 52 due to AA fire and one in the accident mentioned above. One crew member was killed, and 28 were declared as Missing in Action.

At 13.48-14.39 bombers of the 2nd Air Division landed in their bases and the crews could notch up yet another successful mission.

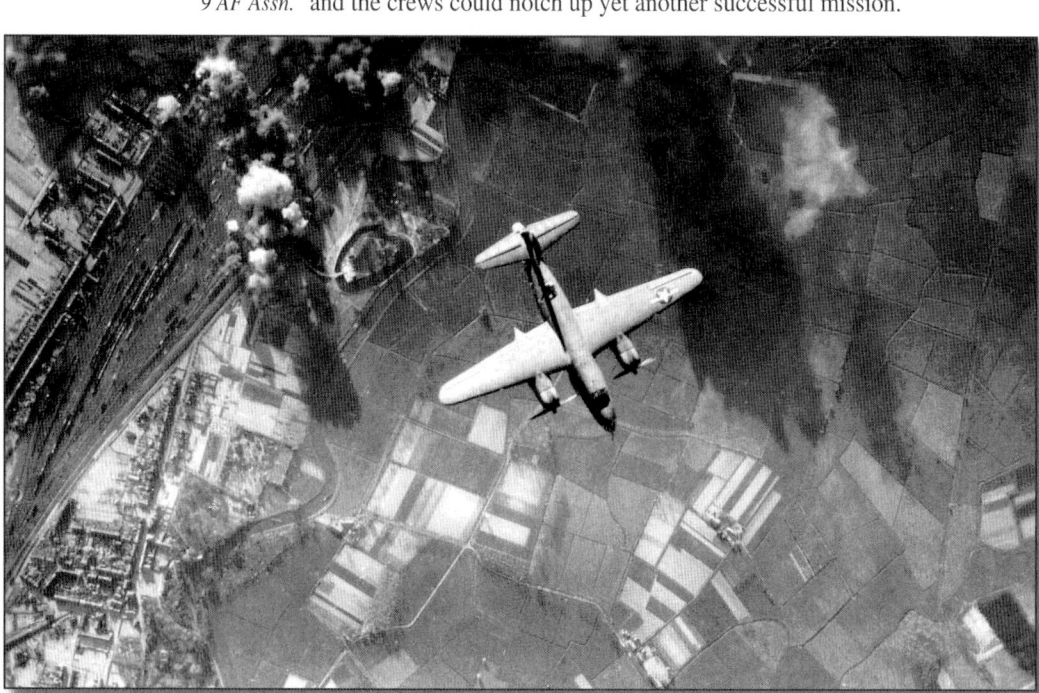

Marauder of the 9 AF during a bombing raid on an unknown marshalling yard in western Germany

9 AF Assn.

9th AF vs I/JG 2

In the afternoon a final action was being prepared that would increase even further the heavy losses of the Luftwaffe and give the finishing touch to the operations of 2 March 1945.

The 9th AF continued operation 'Clarion' that had started on 22 February 1945 and was supposed to paralyse German transport and communication systems. A total of 271 medium bombers took off before midday and dropped 435 tonnes of bombs on their targets. In the afternoon, refuelled and rearmed, the crews were called to action again. A total of 216 bombers took off from their bases and dropped 400 tonnes of bombs on the pre-assigned targets. Bombers of the 8th and 9th AFs were protected by a total of over 1,700 fighters who, apart from the escorting, also attacked their targets, flew armed reconnaissance sorties and patrols, and supported the American 3rd Armored Division in its advance towards the bridge on the river Erft. In a similar manner, support was provided to the XVI and XII Corps in the areas of Sevelen, Mönchen-Gladbach and Neuss, and to the VIII, XII and XX Corps east of the rivers Prum and Kyll, and in the Trier-Saarburg area.

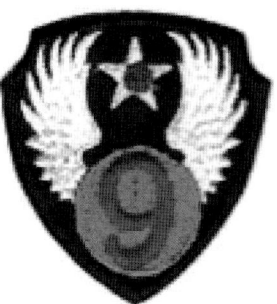

Insignia of 9th AF.

Before midday 40 Douglas A-20 Havocs from the 410 Bomb Group 97 Bomb Wing 9th AF attacked the railway hub station at Simmerdorf and dropped 224 general purpose bombs (56.00 tonnes) on the target. Three machines were heavily damaged by Flak, and 12 more were slightly damaged.

The 98th Bomb Wing with Martin B-26 Marauders undertook a number of actions. The 323 BG attacked two targets. 15 bombers attacked the rail bridge at Eller, but due to heavy cloud cover no results were seen. In the afternoon another 33 machines were scheduled to attack the rail bridge at Sinzig. The other action was a complete failure, though. The leading ship was hit by Flak and was forced to jettison its bombs. The remaining crews saw this as a signal to release their bombs, so they opened their bomb bays and dropped their load. This happened 6 miles (9 km) before the target.

The 1st Pathfinder Squadron led 30 Martin B-26 Marauders from the 394 BG 98 BW to attack a Wehrmacht ordnance depot near Giesen and marshalling yard at Iserlohn. The bombers dropped 59.5 tonnes of explosives on the depot. At 17.22, immediately prior to arrival over the target, the formation was attacked by Flak and over the target American aircraft were attacked by a group of 9-12 Fw 190s and Bf 109s[34]. It can be said for certain that the Marauders were intercepted by I/JG 2 'Richthofen' under Hptm. Franz Hrdlicka. German pilots in their Fw 190D-9s engaged American bombers over Mainz. According to the testimony of the bomber pilots, German pilots attacked very aggressively head-on and from the sides, and they flew in pairs. They managed to shoot down one Marauder, the B-26B 42-95933 'Hillmam Hellcat' from the 1st PFS[35], flown by Capt. P. H. Jones. Fw 190 pilots hit the starboard engine and the crew had to bale out of the damaged machine. The crew included, apart from the pilot, 2/Lt R. L. Richmond, 2/Lt J. M. J. LeBoeuf, S/Sgt W. D. Deoew, T/Sgt H. M. Isenberg and S/Sgt R. H. Felsom. The other damaged machine was from the 394 BG. It forced-landed near Verdun, in friendly territory.

[34] There is no more detailed information about the presence of the Bf 109s. IV/JG 53 claimed one P-47 destroyed in the morning (see the annex). It is quite possible that the IV/JG 53 pilots took part in combat against the fighter escort of the Marauders. This must have been present, as two I/JG 2 machines fell to P-38 and P-47 fighters.

[35] Upon return to base three more were written-off, and 15 machines were damaged. Most of these fell to Flak.

An Ordinary Day in 1945

[36] At the time the 9th AF had two units equipped with P-38 Lightnings: the 370 FG (in early March this was disbanded and converted to Mustangs) and the 474 FG that continued to fly within the 9th AF until the end of WWII.

[37] By this claim 1/Lt Franklin Rose Jr. from 354 FG started his career to become an ace at the end of the WWII. Double claims on 21 and 22 March 1945 gave him a total of five victories in WWII.

[38] That day the 9th AF recorded over 1,700 fighter sorties, losing 1 P-51D, 4 P-47Ds and 2 P-38Js. As the claims filed by pilots of JG 2 are not known, it is not clear whether this took place in this combat or not.

The Germans suffered many more losses than they caused. At 17.30 Ofw. Harald Butter was shot down over Niederwells. His 'Dora 9' W. Nr. 600140 was disposed of by a Lightning[36]. The German pilot baled out but was injured. Ogefr. Herbert Hanck fell to an American Thunderbolt northeast of Mannheim. The pilot was killed. Obfhr. Werner Stempel from 1 Staffel JG 2 was killed in combat over Mainz. His Fw 190D-9 W.Nr. 500393 crashed into the bank of the river Lahn. Recovered from the wreckage, the pilot was buried at Stockhausen cemetery, some 13 km west of Wetzlar.

Uffz. Hans Arck (born on 19 February 1923 at Bonn) and Uffz. Franz Brejl lost their lives over Wiesbaden-Ebenheim and Mainz-Gosenheim. Both these pilots failed to bale out of their bullet-riddled Fw 190D-9s. 3/JG 2 lost also Fw 190D-9 W.Nr. 500072 in combat, its remains falling at Mainz-Mombach. German historian W. Girbig and John Manrho from the Netherlands have independently quoted also the loss of Oblt. Karl Hertl from I/JG 2 that day. Even if archival materials do not confirm this, it is not impossible that he piloted the last mentioned machine. After a combat with superior number of Thunderbolts, Hertl baled out of his damaged machine with his leg shot through, his arm bleeding and with many bruises.

353 FS 354 FG provided one of the groups that escorted Marauders that day. Maj. Delglish led 16 P-51s to protect the B-26s. On their way back two flights spotted ten Fw 190s in the Kirchberg area. They attacked, and as a result 1/Lt Franklin Rose Jr.[37] claimed an Fw 190 at 16.50. It is possible that one of the missing I/JG 2 pilots was his victim.

Oddly, Kenn Rust's 9th AF book mentions no fighter escort. Also other official materials make no reference to its presence[38]. The only explanation of the P-47s and P-38s engaged in combat with JG 2 is that the American fighter pilots attacking ground targets were called to the rescue by bomber crews and wasted no time in doing so.

Interestingly, bomber gunners claimed three German fighters destroyed and five more damaged: a rather reasonable number, compared to the losses of JG 2 and to the 'standard' of triple overclaiming of four-engined bomber gunners.

Participation of III Gruppe JG 2 in the encounter has not been confirmed. However, it lost two Fw 190D-9s due to taxiing and landing errors at Babenhausen, one pilot being killed.

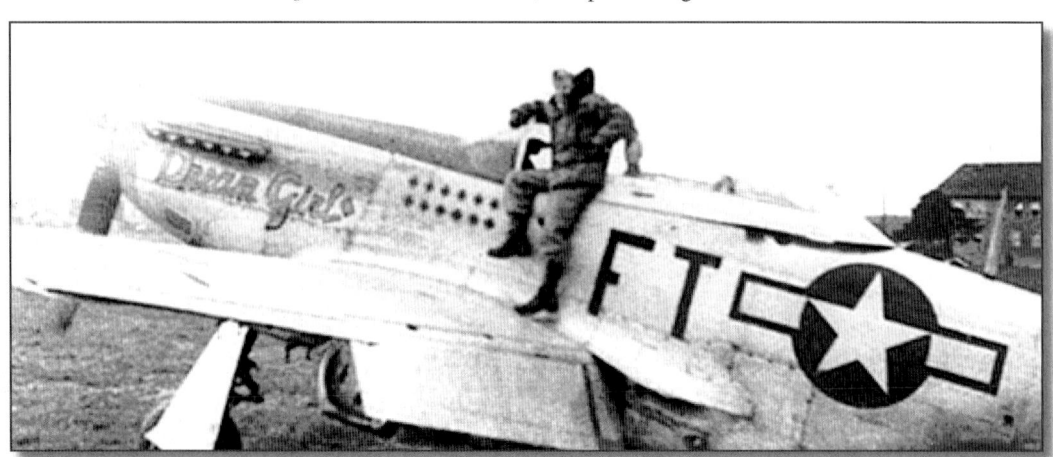

1/Lt. Franklin Rose, 353 FS, 354 FG, 9 AF and his P-51 "Dream Girl". Rose claimed one FW 190 in late afternoon on March 2, 1945, probably from I./ JG 2.
via J. Sterling

This was the end of 2 March 1945. A bloody day in terms of air combat in the European sky and a crucial day for a number of airmen. The Luftwaffe lost in combat a lot of material that would be hard to replace in the fight that was nearly over. The loss of equipment would not be that bad, but the deaths and injuries of the young pilots constituted a marked blow. This was a serious wound in the Reich Defence system, one that would not heal. That was why this was one of the last days when numerous Reichsverteidigung fighter formations appeared in the air to face the Allied bombers and their fighter escorts. The end of the Luftwaffe and of the Third Reich was imminent …

Annex

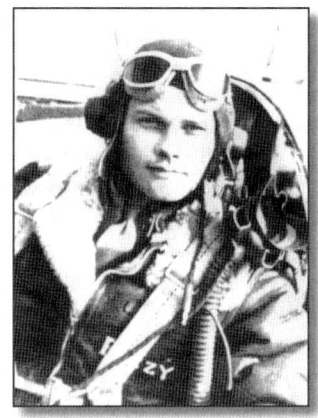

Capt. Roscoe J. Fussel, led the 355 FG mission on March 2, 1945.

via K. Wells

This part serves to provide information about other air events on 2 March 1945 and the remaining activity in the air over west and central Europe.

In the morning of 2 March 1945 Ju 87D-5s from NSGr 1 were engaged by a P-61A-5NO from the 422 NFS 9th TAC. At 04.57-05.06 in the areas F-4067 and F-3062 near Rheine two Ju 87s were claimed destroyed by the crew of pilot 1/Lt Herman Elliot Ernst and radar operator 1/Lt Edward H. Kopsel, flying P-61A-5NO 42-5543. German sources mention the loss of four Ju 87D-5s of the NSGr 1. Fw. Günther Hollwitz and Fw. Herbert Kalb in W.Nr. 142089 were killed, as were Uffz. Paulus Handschuh and Ogefr. Helmut Dehnert in W.Nr.141354. Of the crew of W.Nr. 142096 the pilot Lt. Richard Leib was killed, while the other crew member, Uffz. Gerhard Lübbe, survived wounded. The fourth machine, W.Nr. 142090, was also destroyed, but the names and fate of the crew remain unknown. It was believed that all these machines fell to AA fire. The area where they were lost, near Elsdorf, is not far from the location where the American crew claimed their victories. Thus it seems most probable that two Ju 87D-5s fell to 1/Lt Ernst. At the same time they must have been engaged by AA fire, and the surviving crew member believed that all the machines were destroyed by Flak.

9th AF losses returns include two missing machines from the 367 FG. Its 393rd Fighter Squadron took off from its base at A-94 (Doncourt les Conflans) for an armed reconnaissance. 1/Lt George Juaire led a flight of four P-47 Thunderbolts. The other unit was led by 1/Lt Fred R. Clement with Lt Ed Fritz as his wingman. The pilots broke through clouds and then Lt Fritz saw the P-47 44-20590, flown by Clement, slide and slice through the machine of the leader (44-20487). Both aircraft crashed near Lauchassee, north-west of Metz.

Lt Howard Cain learned about the tragedy on the radio, and flew to that area hoping to see signs of life there, but in vain. Lt Clement is buried at a private cemetery in the state of Maine, USA, while Lt Juaire is buried in the American cemetery at Val du Scheid in Luxembourg (plot D, row 9, grave 13).

The loss of two P-38J Lightnings (nos. 44-23589 and 42-104333) was recorded by the 9th AF during the operation of the 428th FS 474 FG. This was its 307th mission during WWII. Eight machines (two flights) took off at 08.44

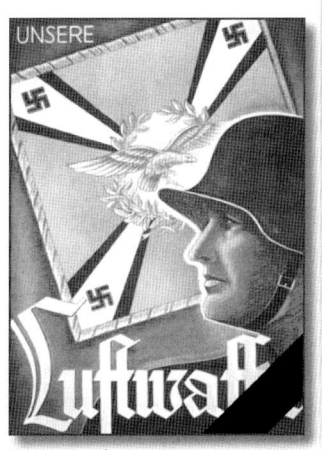

Propaganda poster.

An Ordinary Day in 1945

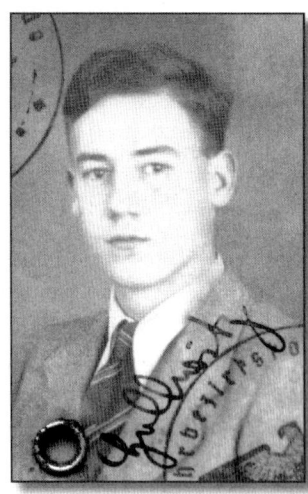

FW. Günther Hollwitz. Born on 15 April 1923 in Berlin Schloßenberg.

from Florennes/Juzanne in Belgium (A-78) for an armed reconnaissance along the route of Bonn-Dresseldorf-Dillenberg-Wetzlar and in the Rhine area. Five machines were armed with two 1,000 lb bombs and three carried two 500 lb bombs. The first flight destroyed a locomotive and eight rail cars were thrown by the explosion onto the neighbouring track. Then the pilots attacked another locomotive and five passenger cars. 2/Lt George W. Alge in his first mission flew as a wingman to the wing leader. He followed his commander Capt. Hanson while attacking ground targets and he was a victim of the shock wave. He crashed with his machine not far from the town of Selters. He is buried at the Netherlands American Cemetery Margraten, Netherlands (plot H, row 4, grave 4). Within a few moments 2/Lt Robert H. Strong who flew as no. 4 in the first flight was hit by Flak. He failed to bale out of his fatally hit machine and he crashed and burnt with it near Mundersbach. He was buried, like his colleague from the 474 FG, at the Netherlands American Cemetery Margraten, Netherlands (plot J, row 16, grave 2).

On 2 March 1945 the 524 FS 27 FG bombed targets in the Homburg area in Germany. The Thunderbolt 'Mini Nr. II' flown by 2/Lt Harold K. Wolf was hit by an 88 mm Flak battery at Kleinottweiler. The spot where the machine crashed is not known. The pilot managed to bale out, but his landing was very hard. His parachute was damaged by rounds fired by the SS unit at Kleinottweiler. Upon landing the American pilot broke his thighbone. He was taken to the hospital at Homburg. During his treatment he suffered from complications and he died of his injuries on 14 March 1945. He was buried on the local cemetery. Then exhumed, he is now buried at the American Military Cemetery at St. Avold, Lorraine.

RAF Bomber Command sent 858 bombers out on 2 March 1945. A formation of 531 Lancasters, 303 Halifaxes and 24 Mosquitoes attacked Cologne in two waves. The first attack was carried out by 703 aircraft and the second by 155 Lancasters. During the second attack, due to failure of the G-H station, only 15 machines dropped their bombs.

The main raid was truly destructive. Pathfinders marked the target perfectly in very good weather. Bombs hit the centre of the city on the right bank of the Rhine. Hundreds of civilians were killed in the attack. This was the last RAF raid on Cologne, as four days later the city was captured by American units. US troops, that entered the city four days later, removed some 400 bodies from the streets. Sirens did not sound until two minutes before the attack. Five bombs hit the police HQ where the local radar station HQ was set up. At least 160 German soldiers were killed there, mostly Waffen SS.

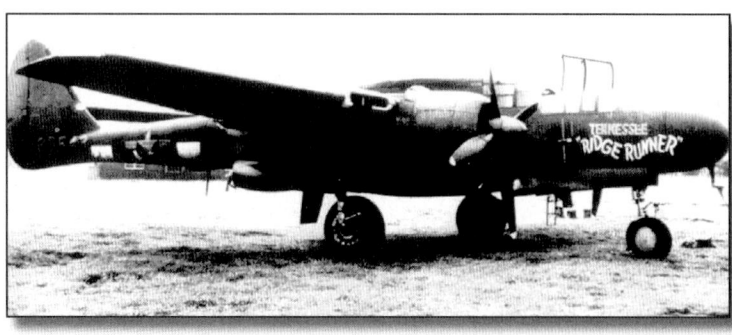

P-61A-5-No, serial 42-5543, "Tennessee Ridge Runner" of 422 NFS, 9 TAC, March 1945.

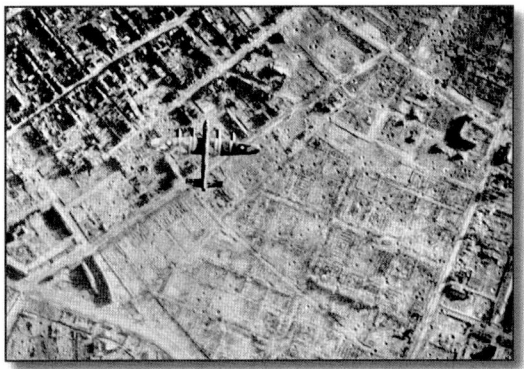 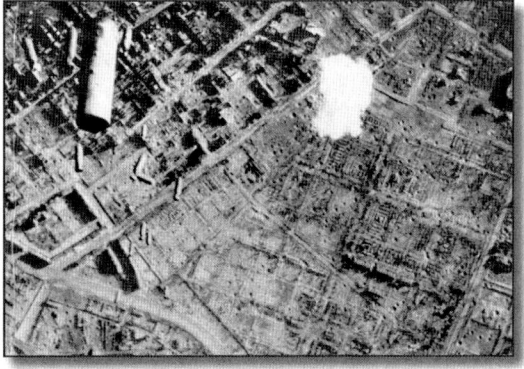

Attack by Lancasters on Cologne on March 2. The leading machine is visible on one photo, and then the others dropped their loads led by the first pathfinder.

Losses included six Lancasters: NN800 PH-A of 12 Sqn, LM723 HW-H (F/O Evans) of 100 Sqn, NG501 BH-I and PB854 BH-U of 300 (Polish) Sqn, RA524 AR-V of 460 Sqn, HK769 GI-D of 622 Sqn, PB158 CF-G2 of 625 Sqn; as well as two Halifaxes plus a third that had to forced-land in Belgium (MZ451 MH-F of 51 Sqn; RG472 EQ-T of 408 Sqn; NP965 C8-Y of 640 Sqn,).

The attack on Cologne involved a Royal Canadian Air Force (RCAF) contribution. 98 Halifaxes from 408, 415, 420, 425, 426, 429 and 432 Squadrons plus 84 Lancasters from 419, 424, 428, 431, 433 and 434 Squadrons RCAF took part. They dropped 1,697,000 lbs of bombs on the target. The RCAF suffered one loss: F/O H. Sproule (POW) and his crew Sgt A. Dennis (POW), F/O J. Moran (POW), F/O V. Mousseau (POW), P/O J. Paxton (KIA), P/O J. Street (KIA), and F/Sgt V. Hunt (POW) flying in the Halifax B.VII RG472 (EQ-T) failed to return after the machine was hit by Flak. Two airmen were killed, five others were captured. It is worth noting that the escort of these raids included 310, 312 and 313 (Czechoslovak) Squadrons RAF. This was within operation Ramrod 1479 and 1480.

The Mosquito of 544 (Photographic Reconnaissance) Squadron RAF with a crew of pilot P/O Ferdinand Kepka and navigator F/Lt Karel Vokoun was sent to a target near Stettin (Szczecin). When crossing the Danish coast the navigator spotted three unidentified aircraft some 12 km behind to port. He gave the pilot a heading south, thus the Mosquito PR.XVI (no. RG 115) flew into the sun. After a moment the navigator lost the unidentified aircraft from sight and directed the pilot onto his previous course. Over Langeland, east of Denmark, the navigator spotted three Fw 190s, one of which attacked from port and behind. The navigator guided the pilot in evasive manoeuvres and led him trying as much as possible to head south, towards the sun and to lower the flight at full throttle, as some 20 miles (30 km) south a cloud formation was present, 6-7/10 stratocumulus with the top at an altitude of 8,000 feet (2,400 m). In a few minutes the intercom failed and the navigator guided the pilot using gestures. Having entered clouds, the navigator tried to fix the intercom, but failed. After they emerged from the clouds they could see no enemy machines, and they flew home.

During the day, at an unspecified time, a Fieseler Fi 156C-3 from 11(H)/12 was shot down with Ofw. Florian Adler at the controls. The pilot is still missing today. Apparently this happened in the area of Danzig-Graudenz. It is not impossible that the Storch was shot down by Mustangs from the Task Force I escort. Mr Slámečka, in his account of the crash of Lt Christensen's machine near Slany, mentioned the presence of a Fi156, and then the flight of a group of Mustangs towards the German aircraft…

At 13.30 19 machines of II Gruppe JG 26 took off from Nordhorn. They flew Freie Jagd north-west of Rheine. The pilots were in the air for 75 minutes without contact with the enemy.

The 15th AF from Italy attacked with 470 B-24s and B-17s, and with escort fighters, the marshalling yards at Linz, St. Polten, Amstetten, Graz and Knittelfeld in Austria, and Brescia in Italy. The bomber units lost five B-24s and a B-17.

The 485 BG targeted the marshalling yard at Linz. 28 B-24 Liberators took off at 09.03. Four machines returned prematurely. 20 machines dropped 40 tonnes of 500 lb bombs on the target at 13.45.

At 12.52 two machines collided, 42-52064 and 42-52644. The pilots Hicks and Lurking recalled: *'I saw both aircraft after the collision. I counted only six parachutes from both machines.'* *'No. 644 slid back, it lost the left stabilizer section. Then it turned up on its right wing and collided with no. 064. One aircraft broke and fell down in flat spin, the other fell to pieces.'*

Eyewitnesses say that they saw six parachutes, but in fact only one of the 20 airmen (both crews) survived!

Both planes crashed half a kilometer from each other, burying 19 men in their wrecks. Because of heavy snow on the crash site it was not possible to recover bodies of the dead until it had partly melted. Magness, Griffin, Jones and Michalaros are buried at Woodlawn National Cemetery, Elmira, NY; Pooley rests at Odd Fellows Cemetery, Danville, Pennsylvania; Fuccilo and Kuszler were buried at Neuville-En-Condroz, Belgium; Krueger rests at St.Avold in France. Lamborse's remains were moved to Arlington National Cemetery and Broker is in Texas, somewhere near his home town of Diboll.

The only survivor, Pilot 2/Lt. Carl W. Langley, was transported to the infirmary at Aibling airfield, where he remained until March 15, 1945.

The third machine lost that day by the 485 BG, B-24 44-40458 of the 828 BS, was flown by 2/Lt Richard T. Loudon who recalled his downing:

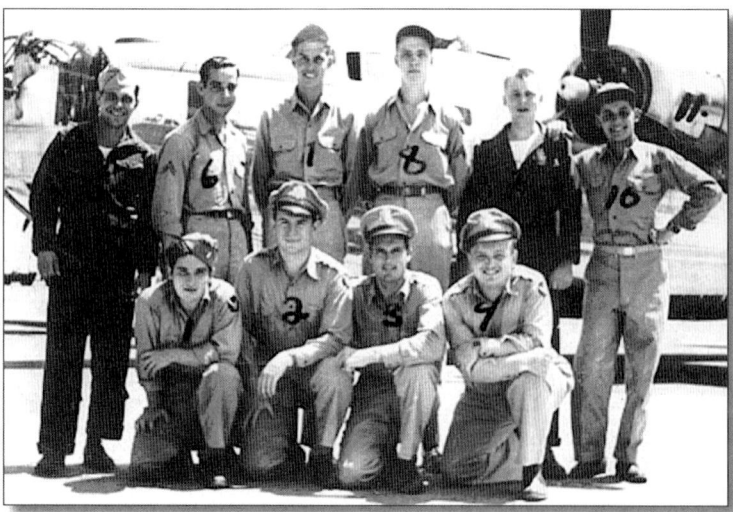

Crew of B-24J 42-52064, 485 BG. Standing (left-right): S/Sgt. W.J. Kuszler, T/Sgt. Ch.W. Jones, S/Sgt. W.L. Broker, S/Sgt. J.N. Magness, T/Sgt. L.R. Krueger, S/Sgt. P.D. Lambros; kneeling: Lt. Carmody, 1/Lt. F.W. Pooley, Lt. Roob, 1/Lt. A.L. Weiger.
via D. Magness

'En route to target engine no. 4 started overheating. I opened fully the cooling flaps, but this did not help. Over Landau, about 3 minutes from the I.P. no. 1 engine became uncontrollable and had to be switched off. Over the target we dropped our bombs and turned back. But without two engines we could barely keep formation with other machines. In the company of a few Lightnings we got over Yugoslavia. The machine stayed in the air with its last effort. When we were sure we were over friendly territory, I gave the order to abandon ship. All eleven of us baled out safely'.

Another machine lost by the 15th AF, B-24H 42-52762 from the 781 BS 465 BG, was flown by 1/Lt Robert E. French. En route to target the bomber was hit in an engine by AA fire. The remaining engines also damaged, the pilot ordered the crew to abandon the bomber. Six airmen baled out immediately and landed at Lápafo, Szakcs, Kocsola in Hungary. The pilot and the co-pilot Kenneth L. Parkhurst baled out a few seconds later. Donahue and Wood were wounded during the jump. Upon landing they were treated in a Soviet field hospital.

1/Lt. Andrew B. Bray, 52 FG.
via T. Tullis

The abandoned bomber continued to fly from Ujregi westwards, made a smooth turn and crashed into a mountain top. The nose part with the wings fell into the valley, while the rear part was left on the slope.

Thirty one P-51s from the 52 FG 15th AF flew on a mission against railway and water facilities in the area from Linz to Regensburg in Germany. As a result of the action two locomotives and two steam ships were destroyed, and 42 rail cars, trucks, cars, a train with a military crew, three factories, six electric lines, and many other buildings and devices were damaged. Lt Bray who participated in the action was awarded the DFC for the results. This is his DFC citation:

'Lt Bray led the flight of sixteen P-51s on a mission to strafe targets along the railroad between Linz, Austria and Regensburg, Germany. Before arriving in the target area the squadron split into two eight-plane formations.

Lt Bray led his flight through the undercast and levelled out at 5000 feet. They immediately encountered intense, accurate, light Flak. Taking evasive action they flew toward Linz and let down on deck as they approached the double-track main line.

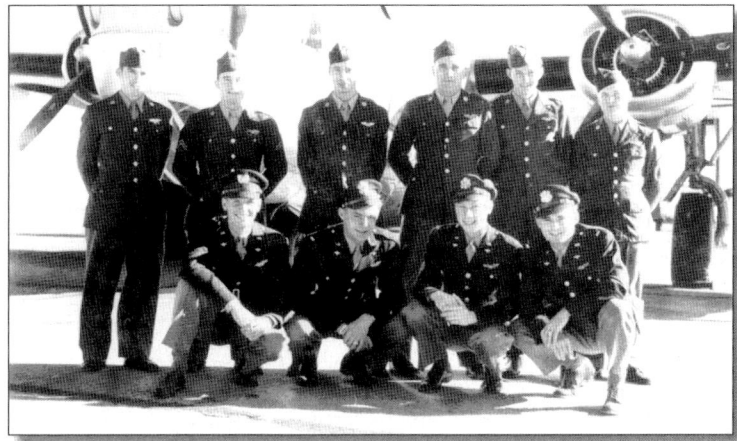

Crew of Robert French, 465 BG, lost on March 2, 1945 over Hungary.

Tálosi Zoltán

An Ordinary Day in 1945

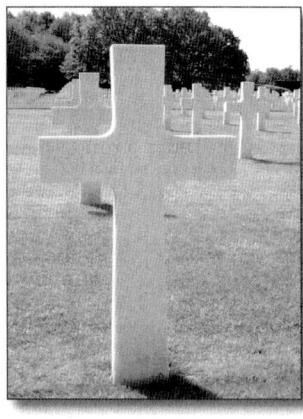

Above & below:
Graves of Allied aviators at American Cemetery at Neupre, Belgium.

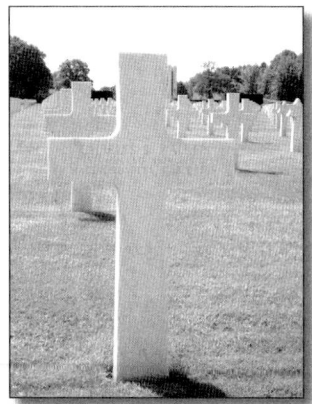

Lt Bray saw three locomotives travelling east and led his flight to attack them. He damaged and disabled the lead locomotive and his flight members seriously damaged the other two locomotives, causing them all to stop; and the personnel to jump out. Then Bray saw another locomotive on a siding with steam up and attached to fifteen boxcars. He fired on these targets, disabling the locomotive and damaging at least ten of boxcars.

Then he saw three Me 109s and seven Fw 190s at about 2000 feet in the Wels, Austria area. Despite his shortage of ammunition after the strafing attack, he headed for the two Fw 190s that were east and away from the other e/a. He approached one of them from dead astern and fired from about 400 yards but saw no hits. Then he fired a long burst just as the e/a started to turn and he saw many hits on the cockpit. The e/a burst into flames, fell off on one wing and crashed into the ground. He then turned into the second 190 and fired the few remaining rounds but saw no hits. He immediately called his wingman to continue the attack but was not heard because the wingman was nearly directly behind him and in a dead area for radio reception.'

Between 08.12 and 09.15 pilots of IV/JG 53 engaged some 30 Thunderbolts in combat. The Americans were probably from the 12th AF. The combat took place over south Germany not far from Schwäbisch-Gmünde. The machine of Uffz. Bruno Hartmann from 14 Staffel was damaged in combat and the pilot was forced to land at Crailsheim aerodrome. The Bf 109G-14 W.Nr. 462798 was 10% damaged. It is quite probable that Hartmann's Messerschmitt was damaged by Capt. Welch from the 526 FS 55 FG 12th AF flying a P-47D, who claimed one Messerschmitt 109 damaged at 09.00.

Later in the afternoon 11/JG 53 achieved a success when Lt. Günther Landt claimed a P-51 at 16.51. This was Landt's 19th victory in the war. It seems quite probable that III/JG 53 took part in the combat with Marauders, or just attacked the enemy that strafed ground targets.

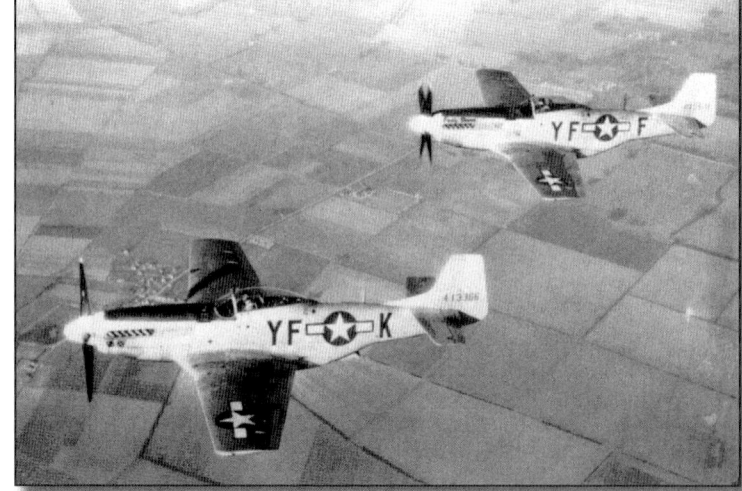

Two Mustangs of 355 FG, 358 FS. Plane with code YF-K was flown by Ltg. William W. Tolby Jr. on March 2 mission.

via K. Wells

In Czech territory an Fw 190F-9 (W.Nr.428443) from a passing II/M Fl. Ü. G. 1 unit crashed. It probably crashed during flight at Podmokel u Děčína and its pilot Uffz. Joachim Kübes lost his life.

The list of German losses is completed by I/JG 77. This was not an operational day for the unit which lost two Messerschmitts during a ferry flight from Beneschau (Benešov) to its new operational base at Prerau (Přerov). Ofw. Willi Hagemann from 4 Staffel crashed his 'blue 3' W.Nr. 512382 (G-14) damaging it 45% at Prerau due to a technical failure. An unknown pilot of 1 Staffel was forced to land due to engine failure in Bf109G-14 W.Nr. 511885 and the aircraft was 15% damaged.

The last recorded activity was probably the mission of 40 Fw190s from NSGr. 20. They attacked a concentration of Allied troops at Goch-Uedem. The thirty eight machines dropped their bombs between 18.45 and 20.43 from an altitude of 700-1,800 m. The return to base proved difficult: two Fw 190G-3s (W.Nr. 160634 and 160072) belly landed at Bonn-Hangelar[39]. The pilot of Fw 190A-8 (W.Nr. 682273) landed at Münster aerodrome due to disorientation.

[39] *Nachtschlachtgruppe 20 was formed on 31 October 1944 at Bonn-Hangelar from III./KG 51, using Fw190F and G versions (losses show that A version aircraft were also used later in 1945). Its one and only Gruppenkommandeur was Maj. Kurt Dahlmann. In March 1945 the Gruppe was located at Gersheim and later at Twente/ Zwolle air bases.*

Sources and literature:

Brýna Zdeněk: *Ješte jednou bratři Preddyové*, APKR č.34/95
Burke L., Curtis R.C.: *The American Beagle Squadron – A Contribution To The History Of The 2nd FS 52nd FG During WWII*, 1st Ed. 1987.
Caldwel D.: *The JG 26 War Diary: 1943-1945*, Grub Street, London 1999
Clostermann P.: *The Big Show (Le Grand Cirque)*, Chatto and Windus, London, 1951
Craven W.F., Cate J.L.: *The Army Air Forces In World War II, vol. 3, Europe: Argument to V-E Day, January 1944 to May 1945*, University of Chicago Press,
Fw 190D-9 a Ta 152, JaPo publ., 1993
Foreman J., Harvey S.E.: *The Messerschmitt Me 262 Combat Diary*, Air Research Publications, New Malden, Surrey, 1990
Franks N.L.R.: *RAF Fighter Command Losses of World War II, volume 3*, Ian Allan Publishing Ltd, 2000
Fry G.L.: *Eagles of Duxford, The 78th FG in World War II*, Phalanx Publishing Company, Inc., 1991
Girbig W.: *Six Months to Oblivion*, Schiffer Publishing, Ltd, 1992
Hawker Tempest: Modelpress
Hess B.: *354th Fighter Group*, Osprey Publ., 2002
Irving D.: *Destruction of Dresden*, Noontide Press, 1986
Kohout J., Květoň J.: *398th Bomb Group a Česká Republika*, Slet Plzeň, 2000
Lorrant J.Y., Frappe J.B.: *Le Focke Wulf 190*, La Riviere, 1981
Messerschmitt Bf 109K, JaPo publ., 1997
Messerschmitt Me 262 "Schwalbe", AJ-Press, 1997
Middlebrook M., Everitt Ch.: *The Bomber Command War Diaries, An operational reference book 1939-45*, Midland Publ., 1996
Moench J.O.: *Marauder Men: An account of the Martin B-26 Marauder*, Malia Enterprises, 1999
Olmsted M.: *The Yoxford boys: The 357th Fighter Group on Escort over Europe and Russia*, McGraw-Hill/TAB Electronics; 2nd edition, 1971
Prien J.: *Messerschmitt Bf 109 im Einsatz beim Stab, I., II. III. und IV. Gruppe sowie Ergänzungsgruppe/Jagdgeschwader 27*, Eutin: struve druck, Hamburg, 1995-98
Prien J.: *Jagdgeschwader 53, A History of the 'Pik As' Geschwader, January 1944 – May 1945*, Schiffer Publishing, Ltd, 1999
Prien J.: Einsatz des *Jagdgeschwaders 77 von 1939 bis 1945: ein Kriegstagebuch: nach Dokumenten, Berichten und Erinnerungen*, Hamburg, 1995
Priller J.: *JG 26: Geschichte eines Jagdgeschwaders: das JG 26 (Schlageter), 1937-1945;* Stuttgart: Motorbuch, 1980
Radke S.: *Kampfgeschwader 54*, Schild Verlag, München, 1990
Rajlich J.: *Mustangy nad Prahou*, in: HPM 1996
Rajlich J.: *Mustangy nad Protektorátem*, MBI, 1997
Reschke W.: *Jagdgeschwader 301/302 'Wilde Sau'*, Motorbuch Verlag, 1998
REVI 24
Richter G.: *Chemnitzer Erinnerungen 1945*
Ring H., Girbig W.: *Jagdgeschwader 27 – Die Dokumentation über den Einsatz und Allen Fronten 1939-45*, Motorbuch, Stgt., 1991.

Rix P.: *Bail Out,* in: Fly Past, December 1985
Rix P.: *My Short War,* in: Combat Report, Vol 1., No 4., 1987
Rust K.: *The 9th Air Force in WWII,* USA, 1967
Shores Ch.F.: *2nd Tactical Air Force,* Osprey, 1970
Smith J.R.: *Arado 234 Blitz,* Series No.1, Monogram Monarch, 1992
The 410th Bomb Group in World War II., Association Press, 1987
Thomas Ch., Shores Ch.: *Typhoon & Tempest Story,* Arms and Armour Press, London, 1991
Young B.B.: *The Story of the Crusaders,* self published, 1988
Ziegler G.: *Bridge Busters,* Acacia Press, Inc., 1995

Archival sources:
National Archives, USA (MACR Index and various MACRs)
Bundesarchiv Berlin (German archive) – Luftwaffe losses, via Jiří Rajlich
Allied and Luftwaffe Discussion Boards – World Wide Web
Claims for USAAF (ETO, MTO) and RAF for 2 March 1945 via Dr F. Olynyk
Encounter Reports for 339th FG via Richard C. Penrose, for 352nd FG via Robert Powell Jr., for 357th FG via Merle Olmstedt,
Bomber Summary, Fighter Summary, Analysis of enemy aircraft encounters, bombing data for 1st, 2nd, 3rd Air Division, Target Assigments, Report of Operations and Operational forecast, all for 2 March 1945 via National Archives, USA
Archív města Ústí nad Labem (Ústí nad Labem city archives), fond Landrát Usti nad Labem, žandárske hlásenia zo dňa 2 March `1945 via Martin Veselý (ČR)
General Mission summary for 339th FG, 352nd FG, 354th FG, 357th FG, 364th FG, 355th FG via Group Historians
Internet/World Wide Web – various sites
The Commonwealth War Graves Commission
125 Wing Operational Record Book, 439 Squadron Operation Log Book
The Luftwaffenkommando West War Diary
Volksbund Deutsche Kriegsgräberfürsorge e.V., Kassel, Germany

USAAF bomber crews missing on 2 March 1945

B-17G 44-6573　　　　　　　　Slaný　　　　　　　　　　　　shot down by fighters
MACR12853　　　　　　　　　8 AF/398 BG/603 BS
2/Lt Donald R. Christensen – pilot (KIA), 2/Lt William H. Love – co-pilot (KIA), 2/Lt Harry Ostrow – navigator (KIA), 2/Lt John V. Gustafson – bomb aimer (KIA), Sgt Robert W. Dudley – top turret gunner (KIA), Sgt Albert S. Carlisle – ball turret gunner (KIA), Sgt Elmer G. Gurba – radio-operator (KIA), Sgt Kenneth J. Plantz – waist gunner (KIA), Sgt Selmer K. Haakenson – tail gunner (WIA).

B-17G 43-37871　　　　*'Perry´s Pirates'*　　　Hradčany　　　　　　　shot down by fighters
MACR 12857　　　　　　　8 AF/385 BG/551 BS
1/Lt Robert A. Krahn – pilot (POW), 1/Lt Oris E. Lundy – co-pilot (POW), 2/Lt Glynn D. Hull – navigator (POW), 1/Lt Russel W. Fritzinger Jr. – bomb aimer (POW), T/Sgt Flem E. Williams – top turret gunner (POW), T/Sgt Paul C. Klinko – radio-operator (POW), S/Sgt Doyle Green – ball turret gunner (POW), S/Sgt Lester R. Brown – waist gunner (evaded) – TG S/Sgt Roy O. Werner, Jr. – tail gunner (POW)

B-17G 42-97979　　　　*'Leading Lady'*　　　Ruhland　　　　　　　shot down by fighters
MACR 12855　　　　　　　8 AF/385 BG/550 BS
1/Lt Eugene J. Vaadi – pilot (POW), 2/Lt Jesse R. Brown – co-pilot (POW), 2/Lt Thomas J. Conway Jr. – navigator (POW), T/Sgt Neil G. Duell – toggler (WIA, POW), Sgt Henry R. Anthony – engineer/top turret gunner (POW), S/Sgt Clarence Arthur Giltz – radio-operator (POW), Sgt Jino O. DiFonzo – ball turret gunner (WIA, POW), Sgt Burke L. Marshall – waist gunner (POW), Sgt Philip P. Penchi – tail gunner (POW).

B-17G 44-8417　　　　　　　　Fictenburg　　　　　　　　shot down by fighters
MACR 12858　　　　　　　8 AF/385 BG/550 BS
2/Lt Kenneth G. Tipton – pilot (POW), Edward M. Craig – co-pilot (POW), Jack M. Waller – navigator (POW), Glenn W. King – bomb aimer (POW), Roger C. Maul – engineer (POW), Frank E. Mang – radio-operator (POW), Glenn R. Jr. Childress – ball turret gunner (POW), Charles C. Eckert Jr. – waist gunner (POW), John Nostin – tail gunner (KIA)

B-17G 43-38148　　　　　　　　Jueledorf　　　　　　　　shot down by fighters
MACR12856　　　　　　　　8 AF/385 BG/549 BS
1/Lt Leon E. Tripp – pilot (KIA),2/Lt Edward L. C. Batz – co-pilot (POW), F/O Edward J. Gildea – navigator (KIA), Sgt Daniel J. Mackiewicz – engineer (KIA), Sgt Richard J. Walters – chin gunner (MIA), Sgt Francis W. Wiemerslage – ball turret gunner (KIA), Sgt Robert J. Macauley – waist gunner (KIA), Sgt Henry Koshenina – tail gunner (KIA).

B-24H 42-51171　　　　*'Eli Swof Jr'*　　　Essen　　　　　　　　Flak
MACR12850　　　　　　　8 AF/467 BG/790 BS
2/Lt Alvah D. Reid – pilot (KIA), F/O Guy F. Shurtz – co-pilot (KIA), F/O Robert F. Herrmann – navigator (POW), Sgt Chester M. Guzik – engineer (KIA), Sgt Joseph A. Dore – radio-operator (KIA), Sgt John T. Watson – nose gunner (KIA), Sgt Bernard A. McGlynn – gunner (KIA), Sgt Benjamin R. Sharkey – tail gunner (POW), Sgt Edward N. Gibbs – gunner (POW)

B-17G 43-37767　　　　*'My Ideal'*　　　collided with 44-8697 over the English Channel
MACR12846　　　　　　　8 AF/96 BG/339 BS
1/Lt Benton R. Gatch – pilot (KLD), F/O John H. Kennedy – co-pilot (KLD), 2/Lt Emmett N. Brown – navigator (KLD), 1/Lt John R. Ozier – bomb aimer (KLD), T/Sgt Loyal A. Bright – radio-operator (KLD), T/Sgt Roy D. Gearhart – top turret gunner (KLD), S/Sgt Robert L. Bashaw – ball turret gunner (KLD), S/Sgt Kenneth N. Bonsecours – waist gunner (KLD), S/Sgt William E. Gorsuch – tail gunner (KLD)

B-17G 44-8697   collided with 43-37767 over the English Channel
MACR12846   8 AF/96 BG/413 BS
1/Lt Herbert E. Stillwell – pilot (KLD), 2/Lt Lloyd R. Snyder – co-pilot (KLD), 2/Lt Arnold Schulke – navigator (KLD), T/Sgt Joel Nussenhoff – toggler (KLD), T/Sgt Hans H. Paulsen – radio-operator (KLD), T/Sgt Ledley L. Basden – top turret gunner (KLD), S/Sgt Herbert M. Lafon – ball turret gunner (KLD), S/Sgt Pat C. Vinzant – waist gunner (KLD), S/Sgt Neil A. Wagner – tail gunner (KLD).

B-17G 43-38828   Bentrode   Flak
MACR12859   8 AF/96 BG/413 BS
2/Lt William A. Hemphill II- pilot (POW), 2/Lt Lawrence D. Van Meir – co-pilot (POW), 2/Lt Raymond B. Baynes – navigator (POW), F/O Alvin D. Murtha – bomb aimer (POW), T/Sgt Arnold Hurst – radio-operator (POW), T/Sgt Ernest Molnar – top turret gunner (POW), S/Sgt Maurice J. Huot – ball turret gunner (POW), S/Sgt Anthony Minkiewicz – waist gunner (POW), S/Sgt Charles A. Krieger – tail gunner (POW)

B-24J 42-51273   Tennenheide   shot down by fighters
MACR12849   8 AF/466 BG/785 BG
2/Lt Howard.W. Greiner – pilot (MIA), F/O Edmund B. Knoll – co-pilot (KIA), Andrew L. Swartz – nose gunner (KIA), Robert E. Shaddy – waist gunner (KIA), Ernest H. Ratliff – tail gunner (KIA), 2/Lt Henry Holm – navigator (POW), Sgt John G. Spissinger – top turret gunner (POW), Sgt Frank J. Korycanek – radio-operator (POW), Sgt Richard Maki – left waist gunner (POW)

B-17G 43-39058   Turek near Konin, Poland   Flak
MACR 12847   8 AF/390 BG/570 BS
2/Lt Richard A. Alberts – pilot, 2/Lt Glenn H. Hale – co-pilot, 2/Lt Robert T. Huber – navigator, Sgt Herman Flax – bomb aimer, S/Sgt Richard W. Laubenstine – engineer, S/Sgt Anthony J. Leone – radio-operator, Sgt Donald L. Hood – ball turret gunner, Sgt Mark Warren – waist gunner, Sgt Lloyd E. Eickert – tail gunner [all safe in Soviet-held territory]

B-24J 42-51302   Detmold   shot down by fire from a B-24
MACR 12854   8 AF/392 BG/576 BS
2/Lt Willis G. Blakeley – pilot (KIA), 2/Lt Harold A. Schoelerman – co-pilot (KIA), 2/Lt CharlesS. Walker – navigator (KIA), S/Sgt Edgar B. Talley – nose gunner (KIA), S/Sgt Richard J. Spades – radio-operator (POW), PFC. Frank A. Amodeo – engineer (KIA), Sgt Robert J. Flosey – waist gunner (POW), S/Sgt John L. Law – waist gunner (POW), S/SgtStanley J. Rubenstein – tail gunner (POW), S/Sgt Herbert W. Halpern – S-27 (POW).

B-17G 43-38102   Trier   Flak
MACR 12852   8 AF/305 BG/366 BS
2/Lt John H. Gordon Jr. -pilot (KIA), 2/Lt Henry D. Newman – co-pilot (POW), F/O Matthew W. Buttiglieri – navigator (POW), S/Sgt James W. Harris – bomb aimer (POW), T/Sgt James M. Simmons – top turret gunner (POW), T/Sgt Byron E. Crun – radio-operator (POW), S/Sgt Peter J. Peck – ball turret gunner (POW), S/Sgt Edgar F. Harrison – right waist gunner (POW), S/Sgt Paul H. Bosworth – tail gunner (POW)

B-17G 44-8141   Böhlen   Flak
MACR 12851   8 AF/305 BG/365 BS
Capt William R. Eyck – pilot (KIA), Lt/Col Howell G. Crank – co-pilot (KIA), Maj Melvin J. Robertson – navigator (KIA), 1/Lt Paul L. Davidson – navigator (KIA), 1/Lt Ira N. Beckman – bomb aimer (KIA), T/Sgt Clarence L. Wheaton – top turret gunner (KIA), T/Sgt George P. Kovalauskas – ball turret gunner (KIA), S/Sgt Raymond G. Pittman – left waist gunner (KIA), S/Sgt Robert L. Lynes – right waist gunner (KIA), 2/Lt Gerald Fitzgerald – tail gunner (KIA), Capt David C. Flanagan – radio navigator (KIA)

B-24J 44-40458   (place unknown)
MACR 12710   15 AF/485 BG/828 BS
2/Lt Richard W. Loudon – pilot, 2/Lt John G. Trieber – co-pilot, F/O Francis Ryan – navigator, 2/Lt Clyde E. Herbold – bomb aimer, Cpl. William C. Washburn – engineer, Sgt William R. Grance – radio-operator, Cpl. Francis A. Rain – gunner, Cpl. Roy L. Wason – gunner, Cpl. Phillip W. Linder – gunner, Cpl. Andrew E. Belloin – gunner, S/Sgt Frederick P. LaPlante – gunner.

B-24J 42-52064   Lanzenkaralpe, Kössen   collided with 42-52644
MACR 12748   15 AF/485 BG/829 BS
1/Lt Earl W. Pooley – pilot (KLD), 1/Lt James Michalaaros – co-pilot (KLD), 2/Lt George A. Fuccillo – navigator (KLD), 2/Lt Albert C. Griffin – navigator (KLD), 1/Lt Adam L. Weiger – bomb aimer (KLD), T/Sgt Lavern R. Kreuger – radio-operator (KLD), S/Sgt John N. Magness – gunner (KLD), S/Sgt Walter J. Kuszler – gunner (KLD), S/Sgt Walter L. Broker – gunner (KLD).

B-24H 42-52644   Lanzenkaralpe, Kössen   collided with 42-52064
MACR 12755   15 AF/485 BG/829 BS
2/Lt Carl W. Langley – pilot (POW), 2/Lt Richard V. Miller – co-pilot (KLD), F/O William J. Hofermeister – navigator (KLD), Col. Paul E. Schutz – engineer (KLD), Cpl. Henry Keprowski – radio-operator (KLD), Cpl. William S. Kaukus – gunner (KLD), Cpl. George L. Taylor – gunner (KLD), Cpl. Doyle G. Summer – gunner (KLD), Sgt Leegrand H. Loller – gunner (KLD), S/Sgt Peter D. Lambros – gunner (KLD).

B-17G 44-6849   Ypps a.der Donau   Flak
MACR 12812   15 AF/97 BG/341 BS
1/Lt William J. Gray, Jr. – pilot, 1/Lt Joseph F. Thomas, Jr. – co-pilot, 1/Lt Herbert D. Bartel – bomb aimer, 2/Lt Irvin S. Taylor – navigator, S/Sgt Norbert H. Moran – gunner, T/Sgt Donald G. Dailey – radio operator, S/Sgt Joseph A. Conway – gunner, S/Sgt Louis D. Persons – gunner, S/Sgt Louis H. Barwick – gunner, T/Sgt Donald W. Carley – engineer, S/Sgt James M. Earle – photographer.

B-24H 42-52762   Ujreg, Hungary   Flak
MACR 12749   15 AF/465 BG/781 BS
1/Lt Robert E. French – pilot, 2/Lt Kenneth L. Parkhurst – co-pilot, F/O David L. Bowman – navigator, Sgt William B. Briggs – engineer, Pvt. Frederick P. Wagner – radio operator, Sgt Francis M. Donahue – ball gunner, Jr., Sgt Denny W. Horton – nose gunner, Sgt Harold E. Quagan – top turret gunner, Sgt Lehman V. Wood – tail gunner.

Abbreviations:
KLD – killed, **KIA** – killed in action, **WIA** – wounded in action, **POW** – prisoner of war.

An Ordinary Day in 1945

503 FS 339 FG mission composition

Bryan	Perry	Gerard	Behrend	Poutre
Preddy	Hill	Terrats	Chetneky	Sams
Butler	Anderson	French	C.Gokey	Frisch
Rawls	Francis	Wilson	Haidle	

55 FS 20 FG mission composition

White	Yellow	Red	Blue	Black	PRU
Gatterdam	Benedict	J.K.Brown Howard		Solmon	Michel
Doody	Fuller	Rackley	Prow	Baker	Chase
Christadoro	Kier	Tracy	Ryan	Peel	
Nauman	Peterburs	Freedman	Skroback		

77 FS 20 FG mission composition

White	Yellow	Red	Blue
D. Van Sickle	Huey	Jones	Larsen
King	Umla	Swierczynski	Drozd
Starke	Pitz	Hall	Cowley
Pierce	Rosenblum	Rege	McCallister

79 FS 20 FG mission composition

White	Yellow	Red		Blue	Black
Meyer	Dufresne	Yarbrough	Bullers		Pollock
Gubana	Jurgens	Bishop		Gardner	Barnard
Ziegelbauer	M. Smith	Schwarz		Pogue	Strock
Stewart	Hennessy	Hahn		Skinner	

487 FS 352 FG mission composition

Halton	Littge	Schuh	Creamer	Stewart	Goebel
Pritchard	Roebuck	White	Huston	Ross	Butler
Doleac	Bateman	Peterson	Miller	Draftz	
Patrillo	Crawford	Vickers	Moats	Thorwart	

328 FS 352 FG mission composition

Duncan	Fieg	White		Middleton	Montgomery
Ridge	Provost	Dodd		James	Owens
Goodman	Cast	Lambright	Camerer	Edelen	
Cartee	Redmond	Rutherford	Price	Sanford	

383 FS 364 FG mission composition

	Hunter	Soth	Couleere	Hassett ?
	Hausenbauer	Gandkaut	Holmes	Jackson
	Kissel	?oodside	Sorrula	Smith
	Cual ?	Hornick	O'Brien	Henley

358 FS 355 FG mission composition

Red	Blue		Yellow
Capt. Fussell (YF-R)	Capt. Blair (YF-G)		Capt. Dissette (YF-Q)
Lt Lister (YF-A)	Lt McCollom (YF-U)	Lt Curran (YF-P)	
Lt Tolby (YF-K)	Lt Allen (YF-I)		

92 BG machines participating

325 BS		326 BS		327 BS		407 BS
44-6948		44-8588		44-8367		43-39048
44-8354		44-8764		43-38962		43-38670
44-8506		44-8436		43-38858		42-97336
44-6559		43-39063		43-37658		44-8612
42-102921	43-39724			43-107181	43-38446	
42-102495	43-39156			43-38675		43-38481
44-6095		44-8764		43-38080		44-8919
43-38401		44-6471		43-39289		43-97336
43-38877		43-37847		43-38477		43-38468

Some serial nos. are incomplete due to lack of clarity in archival materials.

351 BG machines participating

42-102955 Lt L. E. Thomson   42-97252 Lt R. F. Brennan
42-97349 Lt J. F. Beringer   43-37512 Lt E. L. Haskins

43-37515 Lt J. P. Adams
43-37862 Lt A. E. Peterson
43-37956 Lt D. B. Drought
43-38116 Lt P. V. Quinn
43-38465 Lt R. L. Williams
43-38666 Lt J. H. Gattens
43-38813 Lt V. J. Westercamp
43-38954 Lt V. A. Hansen
43-39020 Lt J. L. Hickel
44-6082 Lt G. D. Russell
44-6579 Lt R. H. Murray
44-6907 Lt R. K. Potter
44-8280 Lt J. M. Smith
44-8374 Lt C. E. Daugherty
44-8412 Lt J. J. James
44-8617 Lt B. J. Maddux

43-37665 Lt J. E. Blaney
43-37900 Lt J. H. Hart
43-37964 Lt A. D. Sexton
43-38130 Lt F. F. Horns
43-38640 Lt W. J. Wefel
43-38753 Lt D. C. Rohr
43-38920 Lt A. A. Nowakowski
43-39001 Lt J. D. Rebo
43-39156 Lt M. E. Bone
44-6566 Lt R. E. Mahnke
44-6610 Lt R. W. Brooks
44-8045 Lt R. S. Parnell
44-8358 Cap. F. H. Wilcox
44-8410 Lt C. H. Sugg
44-8468 Cap. E. A. Poston

486 BG Mission #156 composition, 2 March 1945

LEAD element:	LOW element:	HIGH element:
#073 McAnelly-Whitney	#035 Smith-Echenroth	#453 Warmack-McNe
#891 McGuire	#034 Mentzer	#009 Thompson
#952 Riebau	#314 Riley	#902 Casey
#9163 Center-Hunt	#8163 Vance	#006 Dolan
#899 von Platen	#059 Shaw	#091 Hunter
#142 Lowrey	#010 Ewen	#849 Seaburg
#983 Schmitz	#007 Ward	#040 Moran
#616 Thomas	#38001 Bunn	#970 Santa Anna
#041 Bedard	#528 Frawley	#580 Newsome
#954 Ellersick	#996 Gibbs	#835 Chase
#246 Walkup	#149 Melahn	#937 Wood
#846 Sill	#856 Jackson	#973 Williamson.
#945 Burns		

Situation of some of the Luftwaffe units involved on 2 March 1945

unit	Gruppenkommandeur	location	Aircraft in use
I./JG 300	Maj. Baier	Borkheide	Bf 109G
II./JG 300	Hptm. Waldemar Radener	Löbnitz	Fw 190A
III./JG 300	Hptm. Peter Jenne	Jüterbog-Waldlager	Bf 109G
IV./JG 300	Hptm. Heinrich Offterdinger	Reinsdorf (near Berlin)	Fw 190A, Bf 109G
I./JG 301	Hptm. Gerhard Posselmann	Salzwedel	Fw 190A/Ta 152H
II./JG 301	Hptm. Herbert Nölter	Stendal	Fw 190A/D
III./JG 301	Maj. Guth	Sachau	Fw 190D/Ta 152H
IV./JG 301	?	Stendal/Gardelegen	Bf 109G
JGr. 10	ObLt. Georg Christl	Redlin/Erfurt	Fw 190A
Stab JG 2	ObLt. Kurt Bühligen	Nidda	Fw 190D
I./JG 2	Hptm. Franz Hrdlicka	Mezhausen	Fw 190D
III./JG 2	Hptm. Siegfried Lemke,	Ettinghausen	Fw 190A
IV./JG 3	Olt. Oskar Romm	Prenzlau	Fw 190A
III./JG 26	Hptm. Walter Krupinski	Plantlünne	Fw 190D
II./JG 27	Hptm. Fritz Keller	Rheine-Hopsten	Bf 109G/K
III./JG 27	Hptm. Dr. Peter Werfft acting Olt. Emil Clade	Hesepe	Bf 109K
IV./JG 27	Hptm. Ernst-Wilhelm Reinert	Achmer	Bf 109K
II./JG 53	Maj. Julius Meimberg	Malmsheim w. 6.Staffel at Huchenfeld	Bf 109G/K
IV./JG 53	Hptm. Alfred Hammer	Stuttgart-Echterdingen	Bf 109G/K
I./JG 77	Hptm. Joachim Deicke	Beneschau/Prerau	Bf 109G/K
II./JG 77	Maj. Siegfried Freytag	Beneschau	Bf 109G
I./KG(J) 54	Maj. Otfried Sehrt	Giebelstadt	Me 262A
II./KG 51	Hptm. Hans-Joachim Grundmann	Essen-Mülheim	Me 262A
Stab KG 76	ObLt. Robert Kowalewski	Achmer	Ar 234B
III./KG 76	Maj. Franz Zauner	Achmer	Ar 234B

An Ordinary Day in 1945

Luftwaffe losses for 2 March 1945 (via Jiří Rajlich)

pilot's name (fate)	rank	Gruppe	Staffel	type	version	Werk.Nr.	code	cause, site, percent of damage
Abel Fritz (†)	Hptm.	II/KG 51	SK 5	Me 262	A-2a	110553	9K+EN	Nijmegen
?		II/KG 51		Me 262	A-2a	110941		forced landing at Mühlheim, 50%
?		II/KG 51		Me 262	A-2a	110516	NY+BR	forced landing at Mühlheim, 20%
Görlitz Günther (WIA)	Fw.	I/KG(POW) 54	3	Me 262	A-1a	110913	B3+YL	Giebelstadt, Würzburg, combat with P-51, 100%
Griems Heinrich (†)	Fhr.	I/KG(POW) 54	3	Me 262	A-1a	111899	B3+7L	South of Würzburg, 100%
Zimmermann Wolfgang (†)	Lt.	I/KG(POW) 54	3	Me 262	A-1a	111887	B3+6L	shot down upon take-off at Giebeldstadt
? (†)		I/KG(POW) 54		Me 262	A-1a	900699		shot down upon take-off by a Mustang
Metzbrand Horst (†)	Ofhr.	I/EKG(POW) 1		Me 262	A-1a	110655	9K+ZU	Diligen
Löfgen Richard (†)	Ofw.	II/JG 300	5	Fw 190	A-8	960522	green 2	Großtreben near Torgau
Nitsche Hans-Joachim (†)	Lt.	II/JG 300	6	Fw 190	A-8	961109	yellow 7	Zöllsdorf *1) (born on 14 May 1924)
Felske Siegfried (†)	Fhr.	II/JG 300	5	Fw 190	A-8	682965	red 8	Annenburg (born on 23 January 1920)
Werner Karl (MIA)	Uffz.	II/JG 300	5	Fw 190	A-8	681495	red 6	Torgau area, engagement with a B-17
Stoll Heinz (BO)	Lt.	II/JG 300	5	Fw 190	A-8	683316	red 3	Großtreben/N. Torgau
?		II/JG 300	*2)	Fw 190	A-8			Torgau
?		II/JG 300	*2)	Fw 190	A-8	682232		Halle
Specht Karl.Heinz (WIA)	Ofhr.	III/JG 300	9	Bf 109	G-10	151005	yellow 4	Bergholz (near Jüteborg), 100% (born on 16 July 1924)
Jenne Peter (†)	Hptm.	III/JG 300	Stab	Bf 109	G-10	151533	blue 1	Schmerwitz near Belzig, 100% (born on 5 June 1920)
Vogt Horst (†)	Fhr.	III/JG 300	10	Bf 109	G-10	151554	white 1	Niemegk near Kranepühl, engagement with a P-51, 100%
?		III/JG 300	*3)	Bf 109	G-10	151081		Belzig, 100%
?		III/JG 300	*3)	Bf 109	G-10	151541		East of Großenhain, 100%
Schmidt Arno (†)	Fhr.	IV/JG 300		Bf 109	G-10	491200	yellow 7	East of Burg, Stresow, 100%
Leppers Karl (†)	Ofhr.	IV/JG 300	14	Bf 109	G-10	151077	black 8	Wiesenburg/Zerbst, 100% (born on 26 June 1924)
Müller Wolfgang (WIA)	Uffz.	IV/JG 300		Bf 109	G-10	490400		Treuenbrietzen, 100%
Kaap Erwin (WIA)	Uffz.	IV/JG 300	12	Bf 109	G-10	150971		Treuenbrietzen, 100%
? (UN)		IV/JG 300	14	Bf 109	G-10	150895		forced landing at Eilenburg, 20%
Lieb Heinrich (†)	Fhr.	I/JG 301	2	Fw 190	A-9	205941		Řeporyje (Prague 5), combat with P-51
Krapp Josef (UN)	Uffz.	I/JG 301		Fw 190	A-9	980169	blue 3	Vrbičany, Kladno district
Schäffer Hans (MIA)	Ofw.	I/JG 301	2	Fw 190	A-9	202371		?
Güttel Gerhard (MIA)	Uffz.	I/JG 301	2	Fw 190	A-9	207193		?
Schulz Günther (†)	Uffz.	II/JG 301	5	Fw 190	D-9	500569	white 14	Třebíč, Kladno district (born on 30 January 1924 at Cottbus)
Rix Helmut-Peter (BO, WIA)	FjUffz.	II/JG 301	8	Fw 190	D-9	500111	red 4	Chabařovice, Ústí n. Labem district

An Ordinary Day in 1945

Name	Rank	Unit		Aircraft	Variant	W.Nr	Marking	Location/Notes
Müller Egbert (†)	Uffz.	II/JG 301	6	Fw 190	D-9	500429	red 11	?
Kropp Walter (†)	Lt.	II/JG 301	SF 8	Fw 190	D-9	500431	red 1	Würkwitz near Leipzig
Gescheidt Walter (†)	FjUffz.	II/JG 301	6	Fw 190	D-9	500419	red 2	Dráždany
Dietrich Jürgen (†)	Uffz.	II/JG 301	8	Fw 190	A-9	206169	blue 10	Fláje, Most district
Heger Helmut (†)	Uffz.	II/JG 301	8	Fw 190	A-9	980582	blue 4	Dráždany – Klotsche
Ehrlich Wolfgang (†)	Uffz.	II/JG 301	8	Fw 190	A-9	206164	blue 9	Torna
? (UN)		II/JG 301		Fw 190	D-9	500560		?
? (UN)		II/JG 301		Fw 190	D-9	600804		Stendal
Hasenkopf Alois (BO, WIA)	Fw.	IV/JG 301	13	Bf 109	G-10	491186	white 9	Zerbst
Zietlow Otto (†)	Uffz.	IV/JG 301	13	Bf 109	G-10	150812	white 11	Burg, 100% (born on 20 April 1924)
Rummel Walter (†)	Obfhr.	IV/JG 301	13	Bf 109	G-10	150787	white 12	Burg, 100% (born on 24 July 1924)
Patek Johann (†)	Oblt.	IV/JG 301	SK 13	Bf 109	G-10	151515	white 5	East of Burg, 100%
Heilberger Vinzenz (†)	Uffz.	IV/JG 301	13	Bf 109	G-10	150715	white 4	Regendorf, 100%
Keil Leo (†)	Uffz.	IV/JG 301	15	Bf 109	G-10	151087	yellow 1	Gut Lüben, 100% (born on 27 August 1924)
Welsch Rudolf (†)	Uffz.	IV/JG 301	15	Bf 109	G-10	151556	yellow 17	Raksdorf (Regensdorf?), 100%
Hornschuh Siegfried (BO, WIA)	Uffz.	IV/JG 301	15	Bf 109	G-10	491240	yellow 6	Burg, 100%
Bleschmidt Fritz (BO, WIA)	Fhr.	IV/JG 301	15	Bf 109	G-10	151621	yellow 8	East of Burg, 100%
Appel Alfred (MIA)	Uffz.	IV/JG 301	14	Bf 109	G-10	610100	red 4	?, 100% (born on 25 December 1919 at Gurschdorf, † Reesen)
Bäcker Josef (BO, WIA)	Obfhr.	IV/JG 301	13	Bf 109	G-10	491152	green 4	Grabow, 100%
Bayerl Arno (WIA)/Otto	Uffz.	IV/JG 301	14	Bf 109	G-10	150745		Hohensalza, 100%
? (UN), damaged machine		IV/JG 301		Bf 109	G-10	491298		Loburg, 80%
? (UN), damaged machine		IV/JG 301		Bf 109	G-10	150841		overturned on landing, Stendal, 80%
? (UN), damaged machine		IV/JG 301		Bf 109	G-10	150781		Magdenburg, 30%
? (UN), damaged machine		IV/JG 301		Bf 109	G-10	150750		Burg, 45%
? (UN), damaged machine		IV/JG 301		Bf 109	G-10	150843		Brandenburg-Briest, 25%
? (UN), damaged machine		IV/JG 301		Bf 109	G-10	491171		Loburg
? (UN), damaged machine		IV/JG 301		Bf 109	G-10	491214	or 491241	forced landing after combat, Loburg, 10%
Brennicke Hermann (†)	Ofw.	JGr. 10		Fw 190	A-8	171176	black 3	engagement, North-East of Leipzig, 100%
Schimmelpfenning Rudolf (†)	Ofw.	JGr. 10		Fw 190	A-8	731763	black 4	engagement, North-East of Leipzig, 100%
? (UN), damaged machine		JGr. 10		Fw 190	A-8	171698		engagement, Delitzsch, 35%
? (UN), damaged machine		JGr. 10		Fw 190	A-8	980173		engagement, Wittenberg, 40%
?	?	Stab JG 2		Fw 190	D-9	600171		forced landing at Niederstetten, 20%
Butter Harald (BO, WIA)	Ofw.	I/JG 2	2	Fw 190	D-9	600140		Niederweis, combat with P-38, 100%
Hertle Karl (BO, WIA)	Oblt.	I/JG 2	3	Fw 190	D-9	500072		Mainz

An Ordinary Day in 1945

Name	Rank	Unit		Aircraft		W.Nr.	Code	Remarks
Arck Hans (†)	Uffz.	I/JG 2	1	Fw 190	D-9	600142		Wiesbaden-Erbenheim, 100%
Brejl Franz (†)	Uffz.	I/JG 2	1	Fw 190	D-9	210200		Mainz-Grosenheim, 100%
Stempel Werner (†)	Oberfh.	I/JG 2		Fw 190	D-9	500393		Mainz, 100%
Hanck Herbert (†)	Oberfh.	I/JG 2		Fw 190	D-9	500097		South-East of Mannheim, combat with P-47, 100%
Nemeth Walter (†)	Uffz.	III/JG 2		Fw 190	D-9	211041		Badenhausen, 75%
?	?	III/JG 2		Fw 190	D-9	601027		Badenhausen, taxiing error, 10%
Hähnel Walter (†)	Uffz.	III/JG 26	10	Fw 190	D-9	400257	black 9:10	combat at 08.00, 100%
Rögele Eberhard (†)	Lt.	III/KG 76	9	Ar 243	B-2	140178	FI+QT	3 km West of Recke, 90%
Sutterlin (BO)	Oblt.	III/KG 76	9	Ar 243	B-2	?		
Stark Arthur (UN)	Oblt.	III/KG 76	Stab	Ar 243	B-2	140166	FI+EY	forced landing at Lippstadt, 40%
Herkner Wolfgang (†)	Oblt.	II/JG 27	6	Bf 109	G-14	785741	yellow 12	2 km South of Steinbeck, 100%
Eidam Karl-Heinz (†)	Fhr.	III/JG 27	9	Bf 109	K-4	332786	white 9	Brochterbeck near Tecklenburg, 100%
Schaffhauser karl (†)	Fw.	III/JG 27	12	Bf 109	K-4	331458	blue 13	near Saerbeck, 100%
Schulz Erich (†)	Uffz.	III/JG 27	11	Bf 109	K-4	334124	yellow 8	near Saerbeck, 100%
?	?	III/JG 27		Bf 109	K-4	332332		engine failure, Achmer, 70%
Stechbarth Manfred (WIA)	Lt.	IV/JG 27	13	Bf 109	K-4	333945	white 17	forced landing at Achmer, 15%
Pölz Alfred (†)	Gefr.	IV/JG 27	14	Bf 109	K-4	332860	black 18	engagement, Ascheberg/Münster, 100%
Nitschke Horst-Günter (†)	Lt.	IV/JG 27	SK 14	Bf 109	K-4	334134	black 12	technical failure and collision during take-off at Achmer, 100%
Sonnet Robert (WIA)	Gefr.	IV/JG 27	15	Bf 109	K-4	334154	yellow 21	engagement, Saerbeck, 30%
?	?	IV/JG 27		Bf 109	K-4	332797		pilot error when landing at Achmer aerodrome, 20%
?	?	IV/JG 27		Bf 109	G-10	490646		collided with Bf109 K-4 W.Nr. 334134 at Achmer, 20%
?	?	II JG 53		Bf 109	G-14/AS	786337		forced landing due to engine failure at Blankenau, 10%
?	?	II/JG 53		Bf 109	G-14/AS	785762		forced landing due to engine fire at Pforzheim, 20%
Hartmann Bruno (UN)	Uffz.	IV/JG 53	14	Bf 109	G-14	462798		forced landing after combat at Crailsheim, 10%
?	?	IV/JG 53		Bf 109	K-4	332693		pilot error when landing at Echterdingen, 10%
Hagemann Willi (WIA)	Ofw.	I/JG 77	4	Bf 109	G-14	512382	blue 3	forced landing due to technical failure, Prerau, 45%
?		II/JG 77	8	Bf 109	G-10	491379	blue 5	near Prerau ?, 98%
?		I/JG 77		Bf 109	G-14	511885		forced landing after combat near Prerau, 15%
?		I/EKG(POW)		Bf 109	G-6	165578		forced landing after combat, Langenlohe, 15%
?	?	II/EJG 1		Bf 109	G-14	464131		forced landing due to disorientation North-East of Wertheim, 30%
Dahlhaus Heinz (WIA)	Uffz.	I/EJG 1		Fw 190	A-8	680744	white 37	forced landing after engine failure 10 km North of Flensburg, 35%
Endress Martin (WIA)	Lt.	Eins. Gr.	EJG 1	Bf 109	G-6	165813		forced landing after combat, Bautzen-Litten, 15%
?	?	II/KG 200		Fw 190	A-8	680524		US strafing attack, Alten-Grabow, 100%

An Ordinary Day in 1945

?	II/KG 200	Ju 88	G-1	714534		US strafing attack, Alten-Grabow, 100%	
?	II/KG 200	Fw 190	A-8	960539		US strafing attack, Alten-Grabow, 100%	
?	II/KG 200	Ju 88	G-1	714908		US strafing attack, Alten-Grabow, 100%	
?	II/KG 200	Fw 190	A-8	730955		US strafing attack, Alten-Grabow, 100%	
?	II/KG 200	Ju 88	G-1	712232		US strafing attack, Alten-Grabow, 100%	
?	II/KG 200	Fw 190	F-8	580971		US strafing attack, Alten-Grabow, 100%	
?	II/KG 200	Ju 88	G-1	714141		US strafing attack, Alten-Grabow, 100%	
?	II/KG 200	Fw 190	A-8	731012		US strafing attack, Alten-Grabow, 100%	
?	II/KG 200	Ju 88	G-1	714414		US strafing attack, Alten-Grabow, 100%	
?	II/KG 200	Fw 190	A-8	739222		US strafing attack, Alten-Grabow, 50%	
?	II/KG 200	Ju 88	G-1	?		US strafing attack, Alten-Grabow, 30%	
?	II/KG 200	Fw 190	A-8	960541		US strafing attack, Alten-Grabow, 10%	
?	II/KG 200	Ju 88	G-1	714804		US strafing attack, Alten-Grabow, 10%	
?	II/KG 200	Fw 190	A-8	173938		US strafing attack, Alten-Grabow, 10%	
?	II/KG 200	Ju 88	G-1	714287		US strafing attack, Alten-Grabow, 10%	
?	II/KG 200	Ju 88	A-4	3808		US strafing attack, Alten-Grabow, 10%	
?	II/KG 200	Ju 88	A-4	2565		US strafing attack, Alten-Grabow, 10%	
Uffz. Krause Karl-Heinz (WIA)	IV/JG 3	Fw 190	A-8	732009	yellow 17	Prenzlau, 80%	
?	IV/JG 3	Fw 190	A-8	730364		forced landing due to lack of fuel, Güstrow, 20%	
?	NSGr. 20	Fw 190	G-3	160634		belly-landing, Bonn-Hangelar, 90%	
?	NSGr. 20	Fw 190	G-3	160072		belly-landing, Bonn-Hangelar, 10%	
?	NSGr. 20	Fw 190	A-8	682273		forced landing due to disorientation, Münster, 10%	
Ofw. Adler Florian (MIA)	11(H)/12	Fi 156	C-3	?		engagement, Banzig-Gaudenz, 100%	
?	II/SG 3	Fw 190	F-8	930837		forced landing due to engine failure, Pinnow, 60%	
Obfhr. Kainzner Herbert (WIA)	II/SG 3	Fw 190	F-3	670382	yellow 3	hit by Flak, Stettin (?), 60%	
Fw. Hollwitz Günter (MIA)	NSGr. 1	Ju 87	D-5	142089		hit by Flak, 100%	
Fw. Kalb Herbert (MIA)							
Uffz. Handschuh Paulus (MIA)	NSGr. 1	Ju 87	D-5	141354		hit by Flak, 100%	
Ogefr. Dehnert Helmut (MIA)							
Lt. Leib Richard (MIA)	NSGr. 1	Ju 87	D-5	142096		hit by Flak over Elsdorf, 100%	
Uffz. Lübbe Gerhard (WIA)							
?	NSGr. 1	Ju 87	D-5	142090		hit by Flak, 100%	
?	I/EKG (POW)	Fw 44		2953		engagement, Lichtenau, 100%	

An Ordinary Day in 1945

4x ?	4x ?	I/NJG 4	*4)	Ju 88		622806		Vechta, overturned on landing, 70%
Renner Alexander (WIA) + 3x?	Ogefr.	II/NJG 100	*5)	Ju 88	G-6	620873		Trnava, crashed due to technical failure, 100%

Abbreviations and symbols:

† – died, WIA – wounded, MIA – missing, u – unhurt, BO – baled out, POW – prisoner of war, ? – no data available

*1) Some sources quote the pilot's rank as *Fähnrich*.

*2) Both these machines were probably from 6. *Staffel*. It is quite possible that in one of these Lt. Stoll was killed, as in some unofficial sources he is listed as a loss from II *Gruppe*, but in the 5. *Staffel*. He probably flew the machine marked 'red 3'.

*3) One of the machines was from 9. *Staffel* and the other, marked 'white 14', was from 10. *Staffel*.

*4) '4x' means the crew included four airmen.

*5) compare *4). Only one crew member name is known.

Victories claimed by Allied fighters pilots on 2 March 1945
8th and 9th AF - ETO

time	claim	location	pilot's name	Group	Squadron	aircraft flown
0450	Me 110 dam	between bomb line and Rhine	1/Lt Herman Elliott Ernst (pilot)		422 NFS	P-61A 42-5543
			1/Lt Edward H Kopsel (radar op.) [0.0]		422 NFS	P-61A 42-5543
0457	Ju 87	between bomb lire and Rhine	1/Lt Herman Elliott Ernst (pilot)		422 NFS	P-61A 42-5543
			1/Lt Edward H Kopsel (radar op.) [0.0]		422 NFS	P-61A 42-5543
0506	Ju 87	between bomb line and Rhine	1/Lt Herman Elliott Ernst (pilot)		422 NFS	P-61A 42-5543
			1/Lt Edward H Kopsel (radar op.) [0.0]		422 NFS	P-61A 42-5543
0740-0920	*Typhoon, Maltese Crosses	E of Oberhausen	1/Lt Paul I Sparer	363		F-6
0740-1050	*Me 262 unconf dest	Kassel A/F (C-2380)	Capt Bruno Peters	354	355 FS	P-51
0740-1050	*Me 262	Kassel A/F (C-2380)	FO O Ralph Delgado	354	355 FS	P-51
0850	*Bf 109	between Pforzheim & Karlsruhe	Clark		111 RS	F-6C
0900	Bf 109 dam	SE of Karlsruhe	Capt Welch	86	526 FS	P-47D
0915	Me 262	S of Dilligen (Y-1599)	1/Lt Theodore Warren Sedvert	354	353 FS	P-51
0925	*Bf 109	Karlsruhe area	?/Lt Van S Brokaw		111 RS	F-6C
1000	Bf 109	SE of Magdeburg	1/Lt Osborn Howes	357	364 FS	P-51
1000	Fw 44	Illesheim A/F (N-9202)	Capt James P Keane	354	353 FS	P-51
1000	Bf 109	SE of Magdeburg	1/Lt Vincent V Zettler	357	364 FS	P-51
1000	Bf 109	SW of Magdeburg	FO James A Steiger	357	364 FS	P-51
1000	Bf 109	SE of Magdeburg	Capt Robert Gustav Schimanski [0.5]	357	364 FS	P-51 44-14334
			1/Lt Dale Ernest Karger [0.5]	357	364 FS	P-51 44-72313
1000	2 Bf 109	SE of Magdeburg	Capt Alva Cochran Murphy	357	364 FS	P-51

58

Time	Claim	Location	Pilot	Unit	Group	Aircraft
1000	Bf 109	SE of Magdeburg	1/Lt Raymond Matt Bank	364 FS	357	P-51 44-15266
1000	Bf 109	SE of Magdeburg	Capt Robert Gustav Schumanski	364 FS	357	P-51 44-14334
1000-1010	2 Bf 109	E of Magdeburg	1/Lt Jay F Marts	505 FS	339	P-51D 44-14239
1000-1010	Bf 109	E of Magdeburg	Capt James Roy Starnes	505 FS	339	P-51D 44-72152 ?
1000-1010	Bf 109	E of Magdeburg	1/Lt John C Withers [0.5]	505 FS	339	P-51
			1/Lt Harry D Ziegler [0.5]	505 FS	339	P-51
1010	Bf 109	Burg aerodrome	2/Lt Richard I Kuehl	83 FS	78	P-51D 44-72146
1010	Bf 109	Burg aerodrome	2/Lt Hubert Davis	83 FS	78	P-51K 44-11557
1010	4 Bf 109	Burg aerodrome	1/Lt Duncan M McDuffie	83 FS	78	P-51D 44-72036
1010	Bf 109 dam	Burg aerodrome	1/Lt Richard I Kuehl	83 FS	78	P-51D 44-72146
1010	2 Bf 109	Burg aerodrome	Lt/Col John Dave Landers	CO	78	P-51D 44-72218
1010	Bf 109 dam	Burg aerodrome	2/Lt Hubert Davis	83 FS	78	P-51K 44-11557
1010	Bf 109 dam	Burg aerodrome	Maj William Houston Julian	83 FS	78	P-51K 44-12136
1010	2 Bf 109	Burg aerodrome	Maj William Houston Julian	83 FS	78	P-51K 44-12136
1010-1030	Bf 109	Dessau area	1/Lt Arthur Collins Cundy	352 FS	353	P-51
1010-1030	2 Fw 190	Dessau area, SW to Halle	1/Lt Arthur Collins Cundy	352 FS	353	P-51
1010-1040	*Bf 109 prob	Wittenberg area	Maj Vic 'L' Byers	351 FS	353	P-51
1010-1040	Fw 190	Wittenberg area	Maj Vic 'L' Byers	351 FS	353	P-51
1015	Bf 109 prob	Burg aerodrome	Capt Foy E Higginbottom	83 FS	78	P-51K 44-11625
1015	Bf 109 dam	Ruhland area	Maj Walker L Boone	350 FS	353	P-51
1015	Bf 109	Ruhland area	2/Lt Garnett Darrell Page	350 FS	353	P-51
1015	Bf 109 dam	Ruhland area	1/Lt Louis William Lee	350 FS	353	P-51
1015	Bf 109	Ruhland area	1/Lt Louis William Lee	350 FS	353	P-51
1015	Bf 109	Ruhland area	2/Lt Roland J Lanoue	350 FS	353	P-51
1015	Me 262 unconf, prob	W of Cologne	1/Lt Floyd T Dunmire	107 RS		F-6
1015	Bf 109 dam	Burg aerodrome	2/Lt Robert F Rohm	83 FS	78	P-51B 42-106789
1015	2 Bf 109	Burg aerodrome	1/Lt Jack D Hodge	83 FS	78	P-51D 44-15187
1015	Me 109	Burg aerodrome	Capt Foy E Higginbottom	83 FS	78	P-51K 44-11625
1015	Me 109	NE of Leipzig	1/Lt John F Duncan	362 FS	357	P-51
1015	Me 109	Kamenz aerodrome	1/Lt Myron A Becraft	362 FS	357	P-51
1015	Me 109 dam	Burg aerodrome	Capt Robert E Wise	83 FS	78	P-51D 44-63208
1015	Me 109 dam	NE of Leipzig	1/Lt John F Duncan	362 FS	357	P-51
1015	Me 109	NE of Leipzig	2/Lt Oscar T Ridley [0.5]	362 FS	357	P-51

An Ordinary Day in 1945

Time	Aircraft	Location	Pilot	Group	Squadron	Type	Serial
1015	Me 109	NE of Leipzig	Capt Paul Robert Hatala [0.5]	357	364 FS	P-51	
1015	Fw 190, long nosed	NE of Leipzig	Capt John 'L' Sublett	357	362 FS	P-51	44-11190
1015	Fw 190 dam	NE of Leipzig	Capt John 'L' Sublett	357	362 FS	P-51	44-11190
1015	*Me 109 prob	Ruhland area	1/Lt William W Gruber	357	362 FS	P-51	
1015-1030	Me 109 dam	20 m E of Magdeburg	1/Lt William M Agnew, Jr	353	350 FS	P-51	
1015-1030	Fw 190	20 m E of Magdeburg	1/Lt Frederick Butler	339	503 FS	P-51D	44-15134
1015-1030	Fw 190	20 m E of Magdeburg	2/Lt William R Preddy	339	503 FS	P-51D	44-11325
1015-1030	2 Fw 190	20 m E of Magdeburg	1/Lt Lawrence Poutre	339	503 FS	P-51D	44-15482
1015-1030	Me 109	20 m E of Magdeburg	1/Lt Lawrence Poutre	339	503 FS	P-51D	44-15482
1015-1030	Me 109 dam	20 m E of Magdeburg	1/Lt John W Gokey	339	503 FS	P-51D	44-15509
1015-1030	2 Me 109	20 m E of Magdeburg	1/Lt Francis Robert Gerard	339	503 FS	P-51D	44-14671
1015-1030	2 Me 109	20 m E of Magdeburg	1/Lt Francis Robert Gerard	339	503 FS	P-51D	44-14671
1015-1030	Me 109 dam	20 m E of Magdeburg	1/Lt Robert J Frisch	339	503 FS	P-51D	44-14118
1015-1030	Me 109 dam	20 m E of Magdeburg	1/Lt Carl H French	339	503 FS	P-51D	44-13329
1015-1030	Me 109 dam	20 m E of Magdeburg	Capt William W Behrend	339	503 FS	P-51D	44-13627
1015-1030	Me 109	20 m E of Magdeburg	1/Lt Steve J Chetneky	339	503 FS	P-51K	44-11623
1015-1030	*Me 109 prob	20 m E of Magdeburg	2/Lt William R Preddy	339	503 FS	P-51D	44-11325
1015-1030	Fw 190 prob	20 m E of Magdeburg	1/Lt Frederick Butler	339	503 FS	P-51D	44-15134
1015-1030	Fw 190 dam	20 m E of Magdeburg	Maj William Elmer Bryan, Jr	339	503 FS	P-51D	44-15074
1015-1030	Me 109	20 m E of Magdeburg	Maj William Elmer Bryan, Jr	339	503 FS	P-51D	44-15074
1015-1030	Fw 190	20 m E of Magdeburg	Maj William Elmer Bryan, Jr	339	503 FS	P-51D	44-15074
1015-1030	Me 109 dam	20 m E of Magdeburg	1/Lt Steve J Chetneky	339	503 FS	P-51K	44-11623
1020-1045	5 *Me 109 (insg: dragon w/red border) uncr	Dummer Lake to NE of Coblenz	1/Lt Roscoe R Allen	355	358 FS	P-51	
1025	Fw 190 Wurtzler	S of Wittenberg	1/Lt Edward J Sullivan	353	352 FS	P-51	
1025	2 Fw 190	S of Wittenberg	Lt/Col William Bradford Bailey	353	352 FS	P-51	
1030	Me 109	S of Berlin	2/Lt Lindsay W Grove	353	352 FS	P-51	
1030	Me 109	Magdeburg area	1/Lt Joseph Schreiber	353	352 FS	P-51	
1030	2 Fw 190	Ruhland	1/Lt Horace Quienten Waggoner	353	352 FS	P-51	
1030	Me 109	Ruhland	1/Lt Horace Quienten Waggoner	353	352 FS	P-51	
1030	Me 109, eliptical wings (Me-309) dam	Osnabruck area	1/Lt George W Jones	339	505 FS	P-51D	44-11204 ?
1035	Me 109	NE of Magdeburg	Capt Donald Charles McGee	357	363 FS	P-51	
1045	Fw 190 dam	30 m SE of Leipzig	Capt Edwin Lewis Heller	352	486 FS	P-51D	44-14896

time	claim	location	pilot's name			aircraft
1045	Fw 190 dam	Zwickau	1/Lt Merton J Stover	352	486 FS	P-51D 44-14911
1045	*Fw 190 prob	Zwickau	1/Lt Merton J Stover	352	486 FS	P-51D 44-14911
1045	Fw 190	Zwebau	1/Lt David M Reichman	352	486 FS	P-51D 44-13979
1045	Fw 190	Zwebau	2/Lt Charles D Price	352	486 FS	P-51D 44-13929
1045	*Fw 190 prob	Zwickau	2/Lt Eugene A Paulsen	352	486 FS	P-51D 44-11633
1045	Fw 190	30 m SE of Leipzig	Capt Edwin Lewis Heller	352	486 FS	P-51D 44-14896
1045	Fw 190	Zwickau	2/Lt Eugene A Paulsen	352	486 FS	P-51K 44-11633
1100	Fw 190 dam	Chemnitz area	2/Lt David F McCallister	352	486 FS	P-51K 44-11566
1100	Fw 190 dam	Chemnitz area	1/Lt Reps D Jones	20	77 FS	P-51D 44-14823
1110	Fw 190	Prague	Capt Lee E Kilgo [0.5]	20	77 FS	P-51D 44-15390
1115	Fw 189	0.5 m NE of A/F, Prague	1/Lt Earl L Mundell, Jr [0.5]	352	486 FS	P-51D 44-14091
1235	Me 262 dam	15 m NE of Frankfurt	Lt/Col Willie Otto Jackson, Jr	352	486 FS	P-51D 44-14709
1650	Fw 190	Kirchberg (L-7750)	1/Lt Frederick T O'Connor	364	384 FS	P-51D 44-14147
			1/Lt Franklin Rose, Jr	354	353 FS	P-51

RAF – ETO

time	claim	location	pilot's name	Squadron	aircraft flown
0715-0915	Fw 190	near Dulmen	S/L Robert Bruce Cole	3 Sqn	Tempest V NV775
745	Bf 109	NE of Rheine	W/C George Clinton Keefer (RCAF)	125 Wing	Spitfire XIV
750	Ar 234	near Enschede	F/Lt D J Reid	41 Sqn	Spitfire XIVe RM885
755	Bf 109	5 m E of Lingen	F/Lt V W Berg	222 Sqn	Tempest V EJ873
0755-0810	Ar 234	5 m E of Lingen	F/Lt George Wallace Varley	222 Sqn	Tempest V EJ882
0755-0810	Bf 109	5 m E of Lingen	F/Lt George Wallace Varley	222 Sqn	Tempest V EJ882
0755-0810	Ar 234 dam	5 m E of Lingen	W/O T B Hannam	222 Sqn	Tempest V NV695
0755-0810	Bf 109	5 m E of Lingen	F/Lt L McAuliffe	222 Sqn	Tempest V NV670
0755-0810	Bf 109	5 m E of Lingen	F/O H E Turney	222 Sqn	Tempest V NV674
800	Fw 190	SW of Rheine	F/Lt Charles James Samouelle	130 Sqn	Spitfire XIV
800	Fw 190	NE of Rheine	W/O Joseph Armstrong Boulton	130 Sqn	Spitfire XIVe
800	Fw 190	NE of Rheine	F/Lt G G Earp	130 Sqn	Spitfire XIVe
800	Fw 190 dam	SW of Rheine	F/Lt Charles James Samouelle	130 Sqn	Spitfire XIV
800	Fw 190 prob	SW of Rheine	W/O J T Turnbull (Aust)	130 Sqn	Spitfire XIV

An Ordinary Day in 1945

time	claim	pilot's name	location	aircraft flown	Squadron	
800	Fw 190 dam	W/O J T Turnbull (Aust)	SW of Rheine	Spitfire XIV	130 Sqn	
800	Bf 109	P/O L Lambrechts	NE of Rheine	Spitfire XIV RM618	350 Sqn	
800	Bf 109	F/Sgt J Groensteen	NE of Rheine	Spitfire XIV RM648	350 Sqn	
800	Bf 109	F/Lt R Hoornaert	NE of Rheine	Spitfire XIV RB183	350 Sqn	
800	Bf 109 dam	F/Sgt E Pauwels	NE of Rheine	Spitfire XIV RB154	350 Sqn	
800	Fw 190	F/Sgt Philip Henry Thornton Clay	NE of Rheine	Spitfire XIVe	130 Sqn	
850	Bf 109 dam	F/Lt R J Netherlands	N of Rheine A/F	Tempest V EJ739	80 Sqn	
1410	Ar 234 dam	F/O R A Carson	5 m E of Lingen, Rheine area	Tempest V NV670	222 Sqn	
		F/Lt George Wallace Varley [0.0]		Tempest V EJ882	222 Sqn	
1725	Bf 109 dam	W/O J A Cunningham	near Dulmen, A.7050	Typhoon Ib MN863	137 Sqn	
1725	Bf 109 dam	F/O P J Spellman	near Dulmen, A.7050	Typhoon Ib	182 Sqn	

15th AF – MTO

time	claim	pilot's name	location	Group	Squadron	aircraft flown
1110	Fw 190 dam	1/Lt Frederick G Straut	N of Salzburg	52	4 FS	P-51
1110	Fw 190	2/Lt Arnold H Sobczak	N of Salzburg, 48-15N, 13-25E	52	4 FS	P-51
1110	Fw 190	Capt Hans M Zachmann	Wels, Austria	52	2 FS	P-51 D 44-15116
1110	Fw 190	1/Lt Andrew B Bray	Wels, Austria	52	2 FS	P-51 D 44-15435
1115	Bf 109	1/Lt Edmund Palczewski	N of Salzburg, 48-15N, 13-25E	52	4 FS	P-51 D 44-13421

Abbreviations:
ETO – European Theatre of Operations
MTO – Mediterranean Theatre of Operations
dam – damaged; prob – probably destroyed
FS – fighter squadron
NFS – night fighter squadron
RS – Reconnaissance Squadron

location:
E – east
N – north
S – south
W – west

m – mile   (1m = 1.6 km)

US losses for 2 March 1945								
			Fighters					
rank and name of the pilot	type	serial no.	code	AF	FG	FS	fate	notes
2/Lt Henry M. Staub	P-51D	44-63285	HL-R	8	78	83	POW	fighters, Magdeburg
Capt. Alva C. Murphy,	P-51D	44-63765	C5-	8	357	364	KIA	Flak, Grobzig
1/Lt Mathew Crawford,	P-51D	44-15161	B6-	8	357	363	KIA	Flak, Creuzburg
	'Joyce/Diane'							
1/Lt Raymond M. Bank,	P-51D	44-15266	C5-Y	8	357	364	POW	forced landing after combat at 10:40
	'Fire Ball'							
1/Lt Roco R. LePore	P-51D	44-14555	C5-C	8	357	364	POW	Flak, Gueterglueck
	'Pretty Pat'							
F/O. Patrick J. Mallione	P-51D	44-14888	B6-Y	8	357	363	KIA	Magdeburg – fighters? Flak, Haseloff
	'Melody´s answer'							
1/Lt Esteban A. Terrats	P-51C	43-25050	D7-H	8	339	503	KIA	probably fighters, Schlanau
1/Lt Bertis A. Conner	P-51K	44-11363	6N-S	8	339	505	POW	WIA, Flak, Mockern
	'Therese'							
1/Lt Harry F. Howard	P-51D	44-14622	6N-E	8	339	505	POW	WIA, Mockern, shot down during straffing after a ground attack
	'Little one II'							
1/Lt Samuel F. Anderson	P-51D	44-13818	CG-B	8	55	38	POW	Mech. failure, Limburg(B) or Limburg/Hahn (N?)
	'Mah Ideel'							
1/Lt John W. Rohrs	P-51D	44-14781	YJ-U	8	353	351	KIA	Flak, Madel
	'Don Helen'							
1/Lt Edward J. Sullivan	P-51D	44-15184	SX-Q	8	353	352	POW	fighters, Niebel
	'Truly Trudie'							
1/Lt Josep Schreiber	P-51D	44-15691	SX-Z	8	353	352	POW	fighters, Belzig
	'Brad's Dad/Li'l Shirl'							
No MACR	P-51			8				forced landing
2/Lt Harold K. Wolf	P47D	44-19595		9	27	524	KIA	Kleinottweiler, Flak
	'Mini Nr. II'							
Lt Coleman	P51D	44-63686		9	354	355		shot down by a US P-51
2/Lt James T. Hamrick	P47D	42-28811	IA-	9	358	366	KIA?	Exploded in mid-air, 10 miles SE of Pirmassens
2/Lt Laurence L. Baptist	P47D	44-19797	CH-	9	358	365	KIA	Crashed and exploded, Flak
1/Lt George R. Juaire	P47D	44-20487	8L-	9	367	393	KIA	Lauchaussee
1/Lt Fred R. Clement	P47D	44-20590	8L-	9	367	393	KIA	Lauchaussee
2/Lt George W. Alge	P38J	44-23589	F5-H	9	474	428	KIA	Selters
2/Lt Robert H. Strong	P38J	42-104333	F5-	9	474	428	KIA	Mundersbach
William B. Dorsman	P-51D	?	?	15	52	2	KIA	Flak, hillside, Welsch area

Bombers

rank and name of the pilot	type	serial no.	code	AF	FG	FS	fate	notes
2/Lt John H. Gordon	B17G	43-38102	KY-J	8	305	366	1 KIA & 8 POW	Flak
Cpt. William R. Eyck	B17G	44-8141	XK-	8	305	365	10 KIA & 1 POW	Flak
1/Lt Leon E. Tripp	B17G	43-38148	XA-W	8	385	549	7 KIA & 1 POW	shot down by fighters
2/Lt Kenneth G. Tipton	B17G	44-8417	SG-D	8	385	550	8 POW & 1 KIA	shot down by fighters
Eugene J. Vaadi	B17G	42-97979	SG-Q	8	385	550	9 POW	shot down by fighters
1/Lt Robert A. Krahn	B17G	43-37871	HR-N	8	385	551	8 POW & 1 EV	shot down by fighters
2/Lt Richard A. Alberts	B17G	43-39058	DI-N	8	390	570	9 EVADED	Flak
2/Lt Donald R. Christensen	B17G	44-6573	N7-X/E/	8	398	603	8 KIA & 1 WIA	shot down by fighters
2/Lt William A. Hemphill	B17G	43-38828	MZ-	8	96	413	9 POW	Flak
1/Lt Herbert E. Stillwell	B17G	44-8697	MZ-	8	96	413	9 KIA	collision
1/Lt Benton R. Gatch	B17G	43-37767	QJ-	8	96	339	9 KIA	collision
2/Lt W.G. Blakeley	B24J	42-51302	CI-N	8	392	576	5 KIA & 5 POW	fire from B-24
2/Lt Alvah D. Reid	B24H	42-51171	Q2-P	8	467	790	6 KIA & 3 POW	Flak
2/Lt H. W. Greiner	B24J	42-51273	2U-N	8	466	785	5 KIA & 4 POW	shot down by Fw190
Capt. P. H. Jones	B26B	42-95933		9		1.PF		shot down by Fw190
1/Lt Robert E. French	B24H	42-52762	T	15	465	781		Flak
	B24H	42-52533	'No love no nothing'	15	465	782		
2/Lt Carl W. Langley	B24H	42-52644		15	485	829	1 POW & 9 KIA	collision
1/Lt Earl W. Pooley	B24J	42-52064		15	485	829	10 KIA	collision
2/Lt Richard W. Loudon	B24J	44-40458		15	485	828	all POW	technical failure
1/Lt William Gray	B17G	44-6849		15	97	341		Flak

RAF losses for 2 March 1945

pilot's name	type	code	unit	fate	notes
F/O C.H. Motteshead	Spitfire XIV	RN123	41 Sqn	KIA	Nijmegen area
Capt. O. Ullestad	Tempest V	EJ691 (W2-L)	80 Sqn	EVD	shot down by Bf109 SW of Rheine
F/Lt G.G. Earp	Spitfire XIV	RM750	130 Sqn	POW	Rheine
F/O A.W. Heale	Spitfire XIV	RM914 (AP-D)	130 Sqn	POW	Rheine
W/O W.A. Livesley	Typhoon 1b	MN354 (TP-K)	198 Sqn	KIA	shot down by US P-51 NW of Neuss
F/Lt D.J. Heard (RCAF)	Typhoon 1b	RB285 'Z'	438 Sqn	POW	Flak, Appelhüssen
F/Lt L.C. Shaver (RCAF)	Typhoon 1b	MN144	439 Sqn	KIA	Flak, NE of Dulmen
McCarthy	Typhoon 1b		44 Sqn	OK.	forced landing at Eindhoven

DRAWINGS NOT TO SCALE

An Ordinary Day in 1945

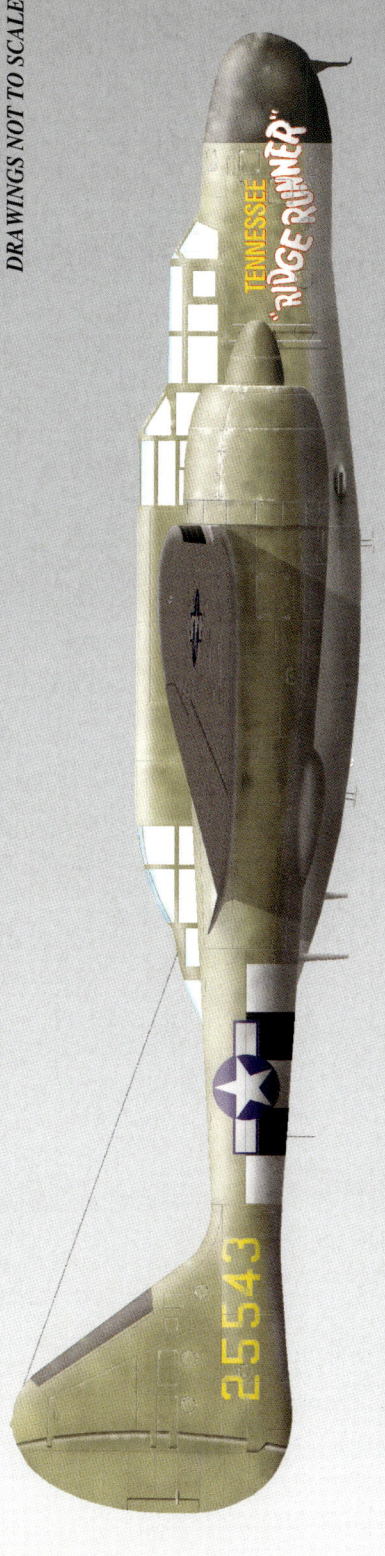
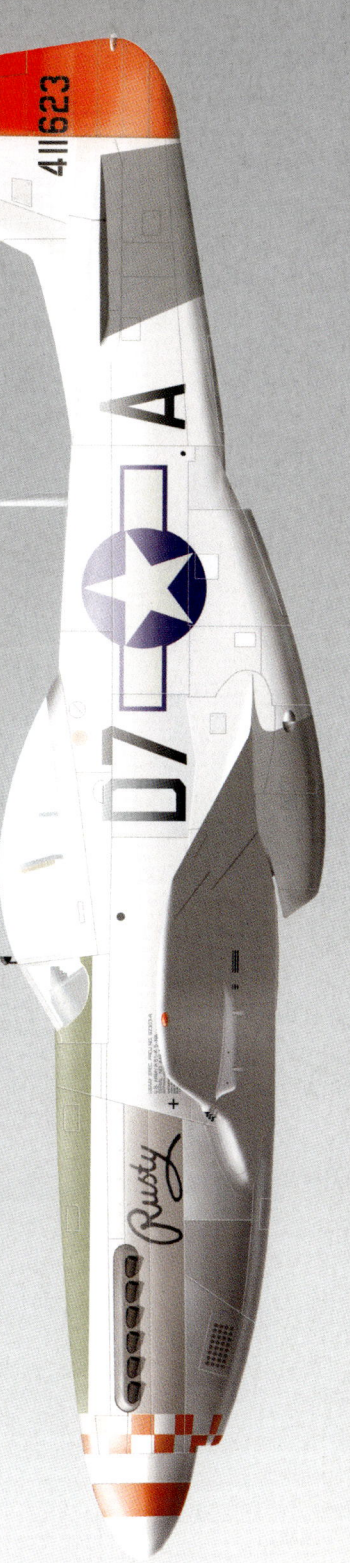

P-61A-5-NO 42-5543 *"Tennessee Ridge Runner"* 422 NFS, 9 TAC. Camouflage Olive Drab/Neutral Grey, nose radar housing black. With this plane 1st/Lt Ernst and 1st/Lt Kopsel shot down 2 Ju 87D-8s from the NSGr. 1 early in the morning.

P-51K-5-NT 44-11623 D7-A *"Rusty"*, 339 FG, 505 FS, 8 AF, 1st/Lt Steve J Chetneky. Natural metal with Olive Drab antiglare panel. With this machine (which had been the personal mount of Capt. Lloyd J French) 1st/Lt Chetneky shot down a Bf 109 and damaged another. The a/c was flown later by 1st/Lt William R Preddy (the brother of the famous ace George E. Preddy, KIA 24.12.1944) and shot down on April 18th with Lt Preddy KIA.

An Ordinary Day in 1945

DRAWINGS NOT TO SCALE

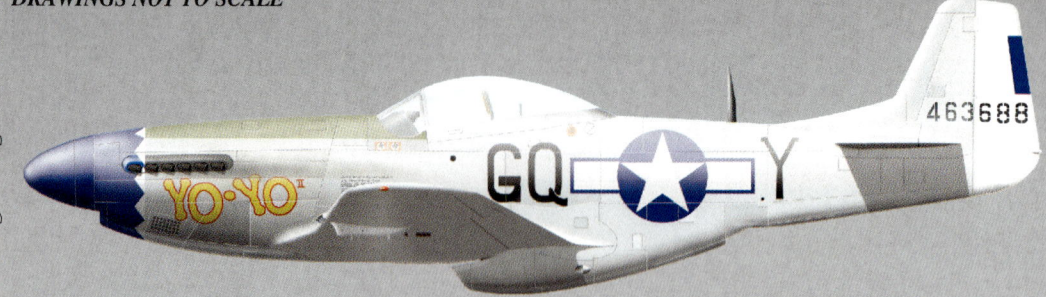

P-51D-20-NA 44-63688 GQ-Y "Yo-Yo II", 354 FG, 355 FS, 9 AF, Capt Bruno Peters.
Natural metal with Olive Drab anti-glare panel. With this a/c Capt. Peters shot down the Me 262A-2a flown by Fhr Griems of 3./KG(J) 54.

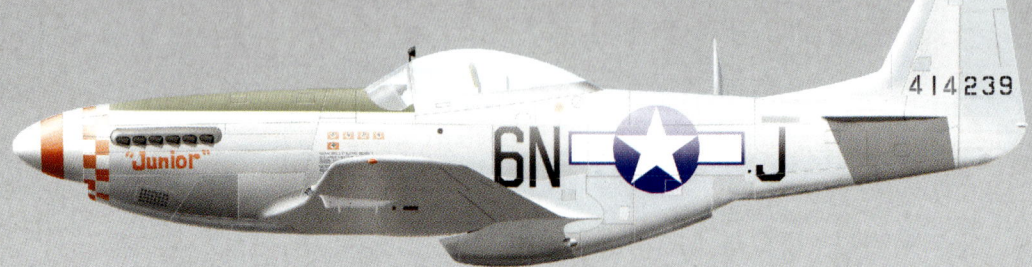

P-51D-10-NA 44-14239 6N-J "Junior", 339 FG, 505 FS, 8 AF, 1st/Lt Jay F Marts. Natural metal with Olive Drab anti-glare panel. 1st/Lt Marts shot down 2 Bf109s of JG 300 whilst flying this machine.

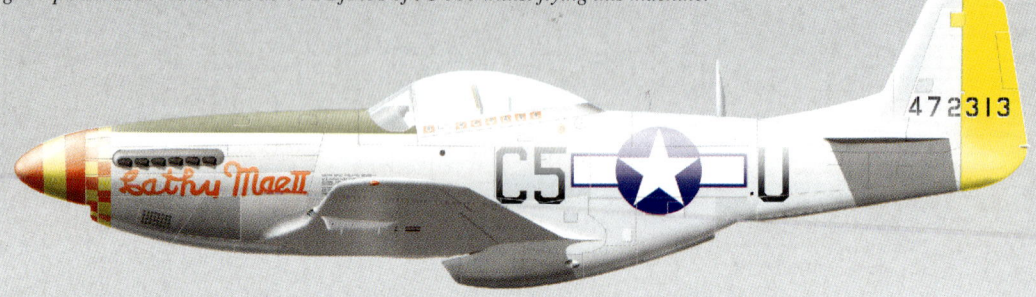

P-51D-20-NA 44-72313 C5-U "Cathy Mae II", 357 FG, 364 FS, 8 AF, 2nd/Lt Dale Karger.
Natural metal with Olive Drab anti-glare panel. With this a/c 2nd/Lt Karger shot down (together with Capt. Schimanski) a Bf 109 and destroyed or damaged several "Mistels" on the Alten Grabow airfield.

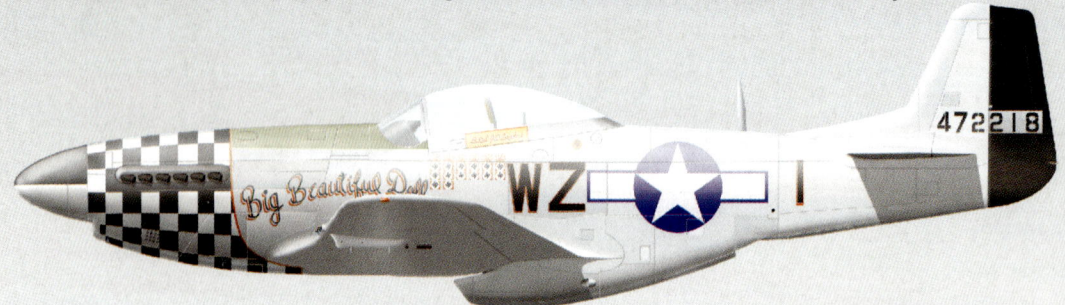

P-51D-20-NA 44-72218 WZ-I "Big Beautiful Doll" 78 FG, 84 FS, 8 AF, Lt.Col. John D Landers.
Natural metal, Olive Drab anti-glare panel, nose painted in white/black checkerboard outlined red. With this a/c Lt.Col. Landers shot down 2 Bf 109s of IV/JG 301.

DRAWINGS NOT TO SCALE

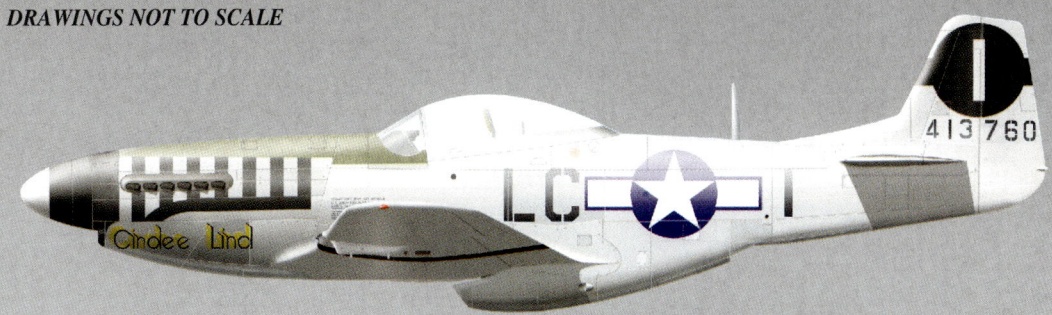

P-51D-5-NA 44-13760 LC-I "Cindee Lind", 20 FG, 77 FS, 8 AF, 1st/Lt David F McCallister.
Natural metal with Olive Drab anti-glare panel. While flying this plane 1st/Lt McCallister probably shot down a Fw 190 (the pilot claimed only damage to the enemy machine).

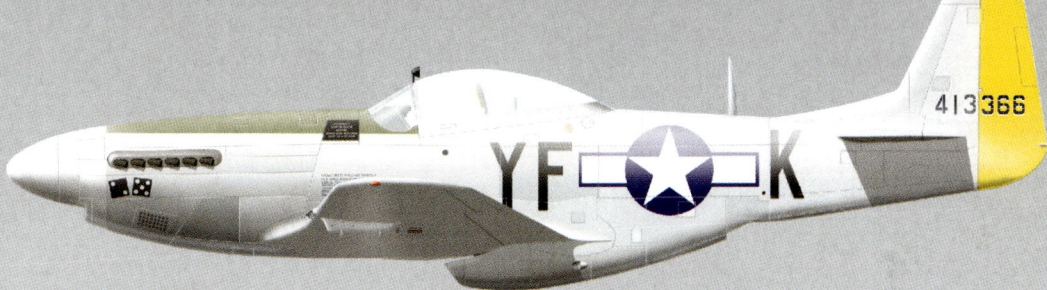

P-51D-5-NA 44-13366 YF-K "Seven" 355 FG, 358 FS, 8 AF, 1st/Lt William W Tolby.
Natural metal with Olive Drab anti-glare panel. With this plane 1st/Lt Tolby took part in combats on March 2nd but without success. Previously the a/c wore the name "Darlin' Marion".

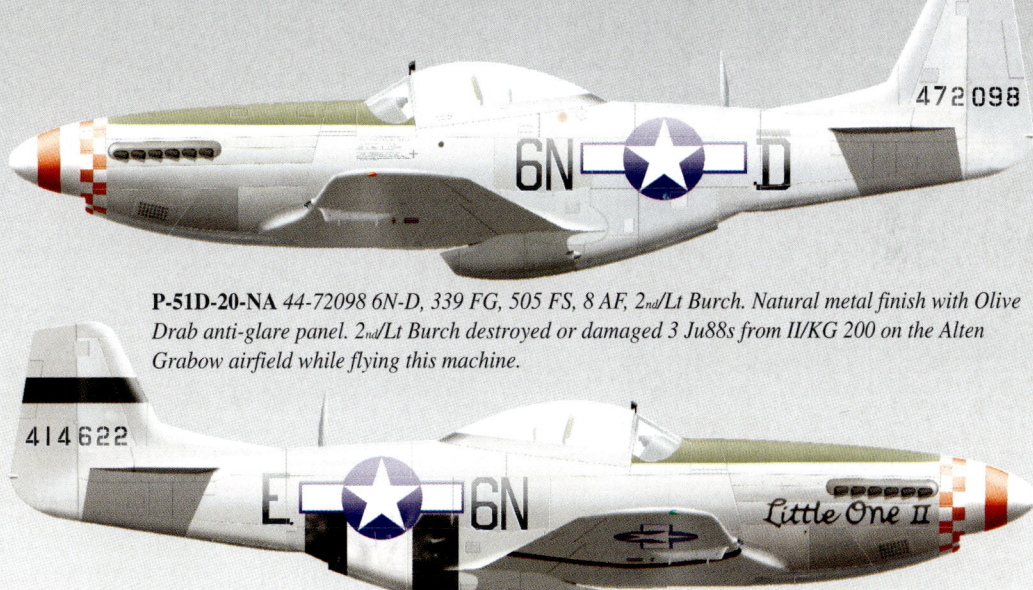

P-51D-20-NA 44-72098 6N-D, 339 FG, 505 FS, 8 AF, 2nd/Lt Burch. Natural metal finish with Olive Drab anti-glare panel. 2nd/Lt Burch destroyed or damaged 3 Ju88s from II/KG 200 on the Alten Grabow airfield while flying this machine.

P-51D-10-NA 44-14622 6N-E "Little One II", 339 FG, 505 FS, 8 AF, 2nd/Lt Harvey Howard. Natural metal with Olive Drab anti-glare panel. This a/c was shot down while strafing the Alten Grabow airfield, its pilot became POW. The plane was the personal mount of Capt. James G Robinson.

An Ordinary Day in 1945

An Ordinary Day in 1945

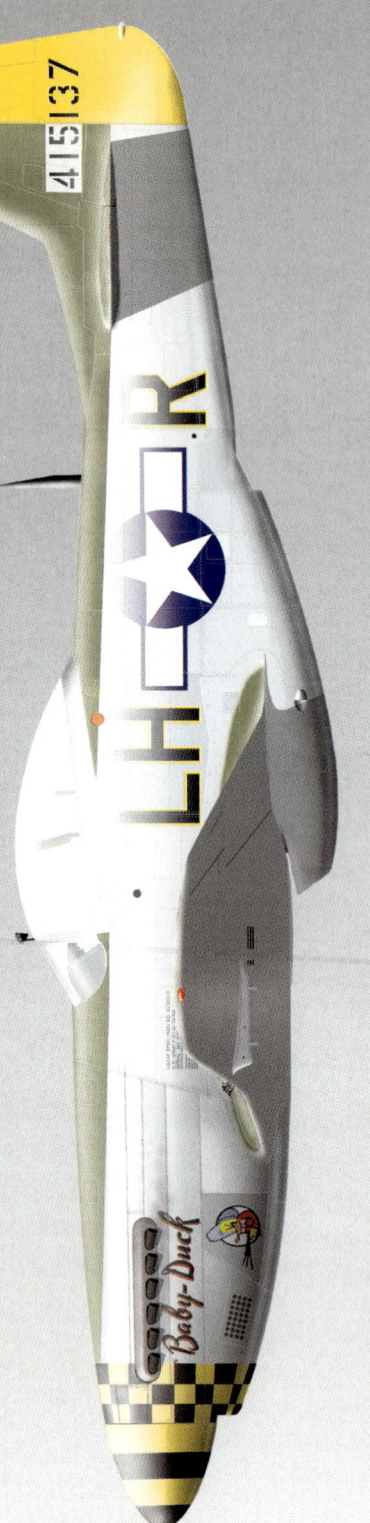

P-51D-15-NA *44-15137 LH-R "Baby Duck", 353 FG, 350 FS, 8 AF, 2nd/Lt Garnett D Page.*
Natrual metal, with upper surfaces painted Olive Drab. With this a/c 2nd/Lt Page shot down a Bf 109. On March 18th the plane was shot down near Berlin by a Russian La-5FN fighter; the pilot returned home safely. Previously this a/c had been the personal mount of Capt. Herbert G Colb.

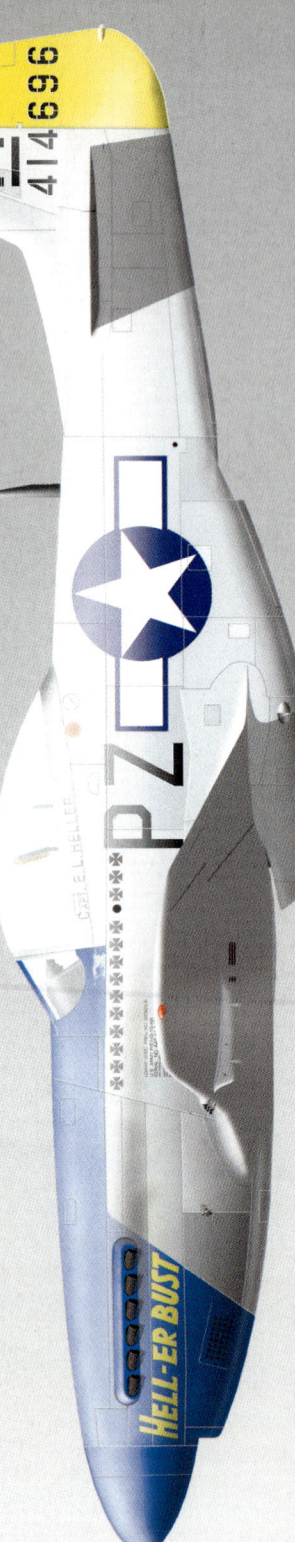

P-51D-10-NA *44-14696 PZ-H "Hell-Er Bust" 352 FG, 486 FS, 8 AF, 1st/Lt Edwin L Heller.*
Natural metal, nose painted blue. 1st/Lt Heller shot down a Fw 190 from III/JG 301 and damaged another one whilst flying this machine. The profile shows Lt Heller's machine in the evening of March 2nd (13 victory crosses).

DRAWINGS NOT TO SCALE

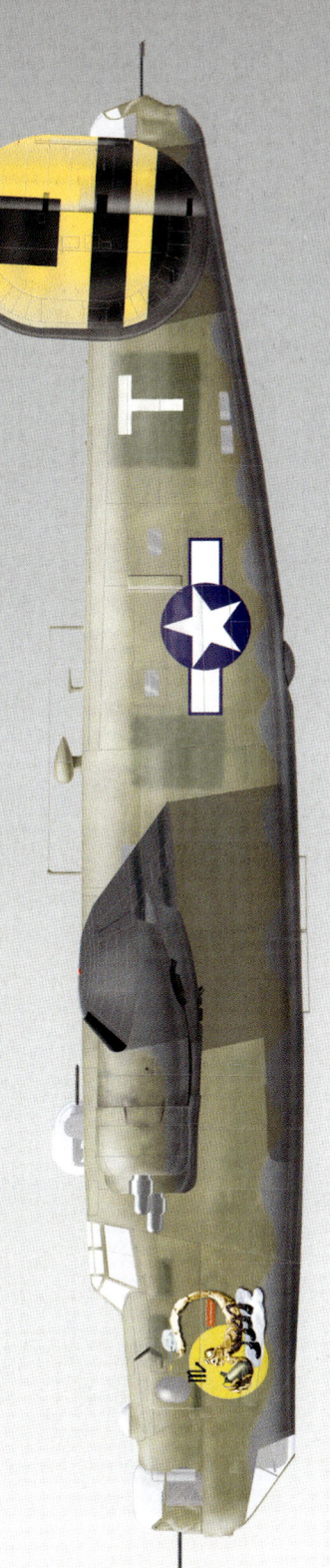
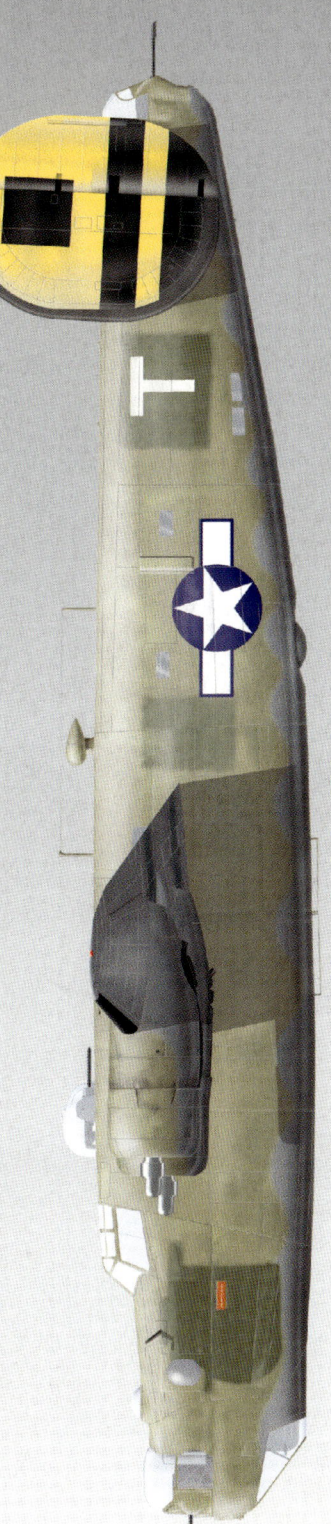

An Ordinary Day in 1945

DRAWINGS NOT TO SCALE

B-24H-15-FO 42-52762 T, 465 BG, 781 BS, 15 AF, 1ₛₜ/Lt. French. Olive Drab/Neutral Grey. The plane was hit by Flak, the crew left the machine with parachutes over Hungary and were captured by the Russians. The plane served previously in the 834 BS, 486 BG, 8 AF, known as the "Zodiac squadron" and wore codes 2S-J and the painting of a "Scorpion" made by Cpl Phil Brinkman. It is not known if the "Scorpion" was painted over while in the 781 BS, but probably not. The camouflage is worn & weathered; previous markings painted over with "fresh" Olive Drab. This is how the aircraft POSSIBLY looked!

An Ordinary Day in 1945

DRAWINGS NOT TO SCALE

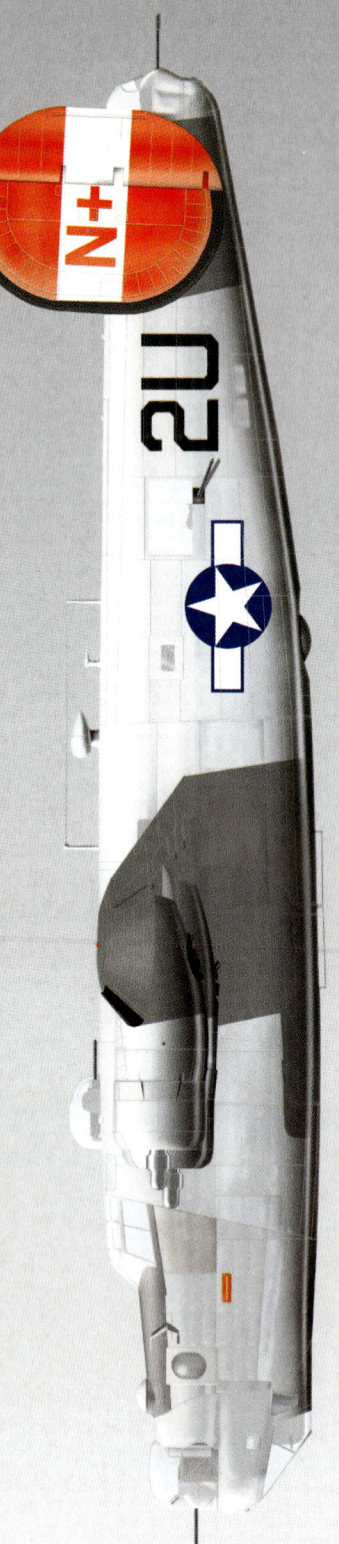

B-24J-1-DT *42-51273 2U-N, 466 BG, 785 BS, 8 AF, 2nd/Lt. Greiner. Natural metal overall, black anti-glare panel. The machine was probably shot down by a Fw 190 and is assumed as MIA together with its crew. This is how the aircraft POSSIBLY looked!*

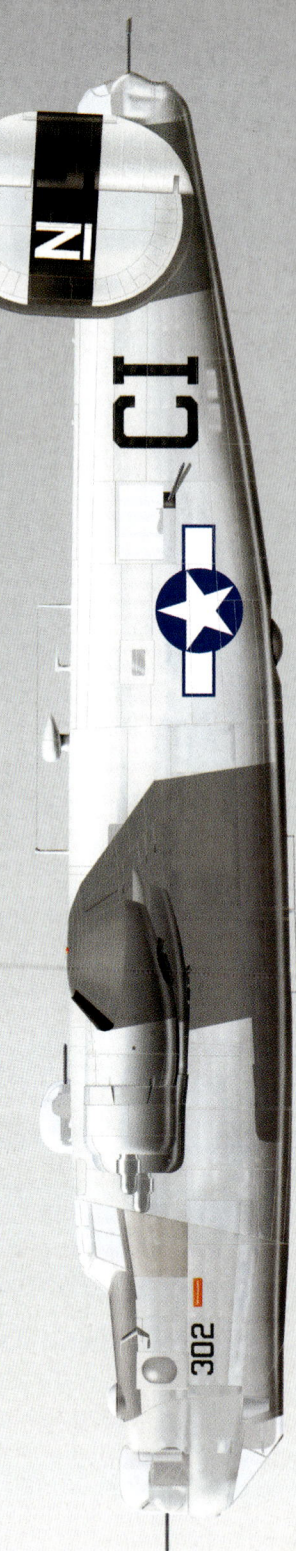

B-24J-5-DT *42-51302 CI-N, 392 BG, 376 BS, 8 AF, 2nd/Lt. W.G. Blakeley. Natural metal overall, black anti-glare panel. The aircraft was shot down by its formation neighbour –B-24 42-29476, which was testing the rear turret machine guns. Five crew members were KIA. This is how the aircraft POSSIBLY looked!*

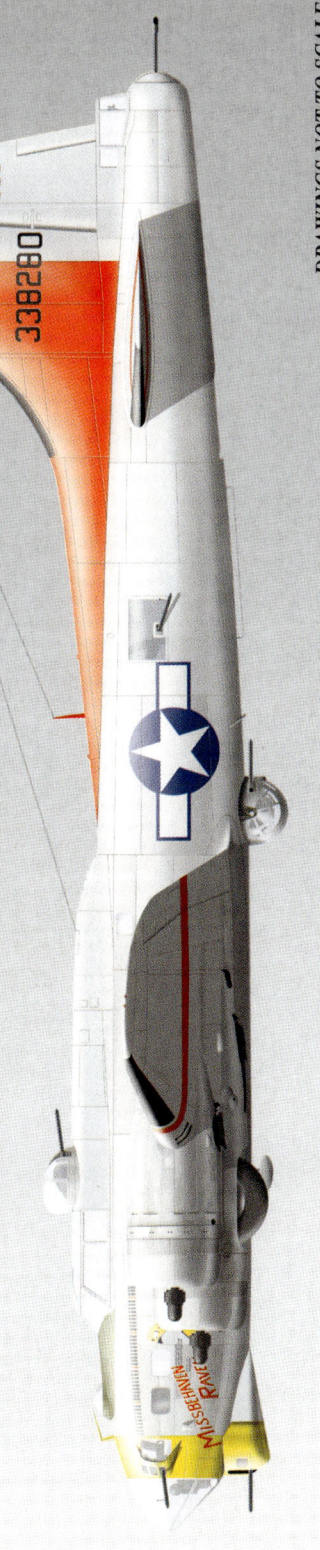
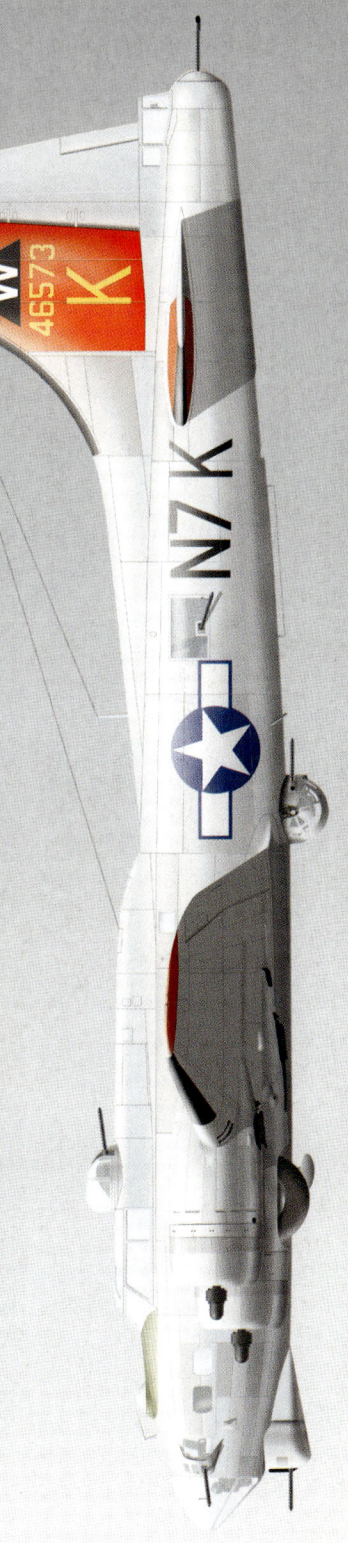

DRAWINGS NOT TO SCALE

B-17G-85-BO 43-38280 (2R)-M "Missbehaven Raven" 34 BG, 7 BS, 8 AF, 1st/Lt. MacTaggart. Natural metal, OD anti-glare panel. The ball turret gunner of this plane claimed one Bf 109 probably s/d. The nose art consists of an inscription, a painting of a strange "bird", and 43 small bombs; each tenth bomb was red, the rest were black.

B-17G-55-DL 44-6573 N7-K 398 BG, 603 BS, 8 AF, 1st/Lt. Donald Christensen. Natural metal, OD anti-glare panel. The aircraft was shot down by a Fw 190 from II/JG 301, the entire crew KIA except rear gunner Sgt Haakeson. This is how the aircraft POSSIBLY looked!

An Ordinary Day in 1945

71

An Ordinary Day in 1945

DRAWINGS NOT TO SCALE

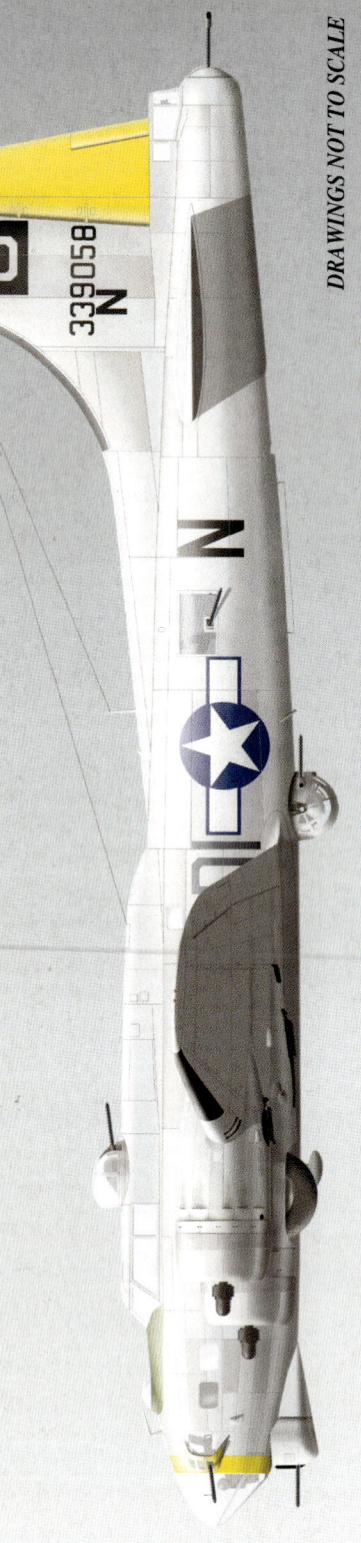

B-17G-100-BO *43-39058 DI-N, 390 BG, 570 BS, 8 AF. Natural metal, OD anti-glare panel. The plane was hit in the No. 3 engine, left the formation and flew east to Russian lines. The B-17 landed in Poland nearby the town of Turek (another version – according to the 390 BG website – has the B-17 crashing in Czechoslovakia near Litoměřice); the crew was captured by the Russians and survived.*

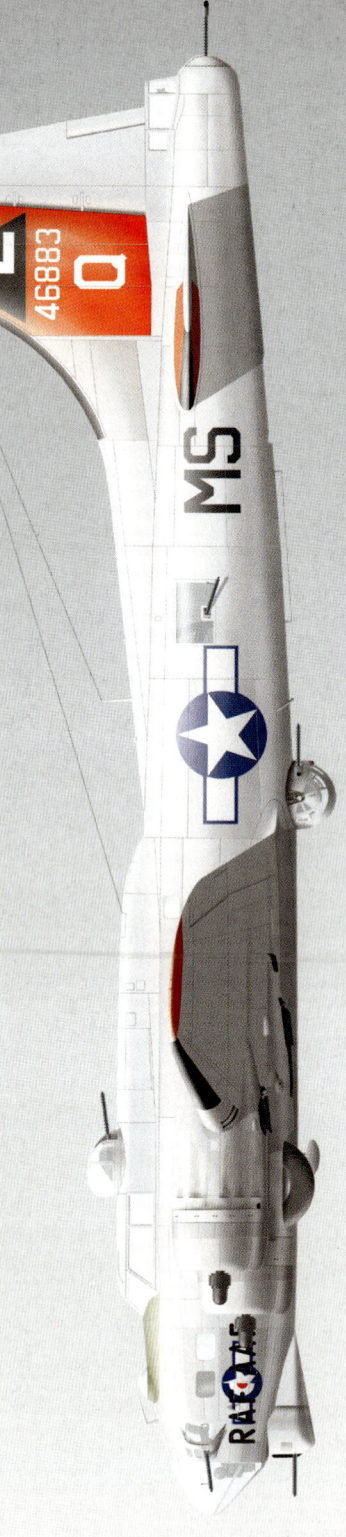

B-17G-70-DL *44-6883 MS-Q "RAFAAF", 381 BG, 535 BS, 8 AF, 1/Lt. Charles Carpenter. Natural metal, OD anti-glare panel. A reserve machine; it took part in a bombing raid against Köln together with RAF Lancasters.*

An Ordinary Day in 1945

DRAWINGS NOT TO SCALE

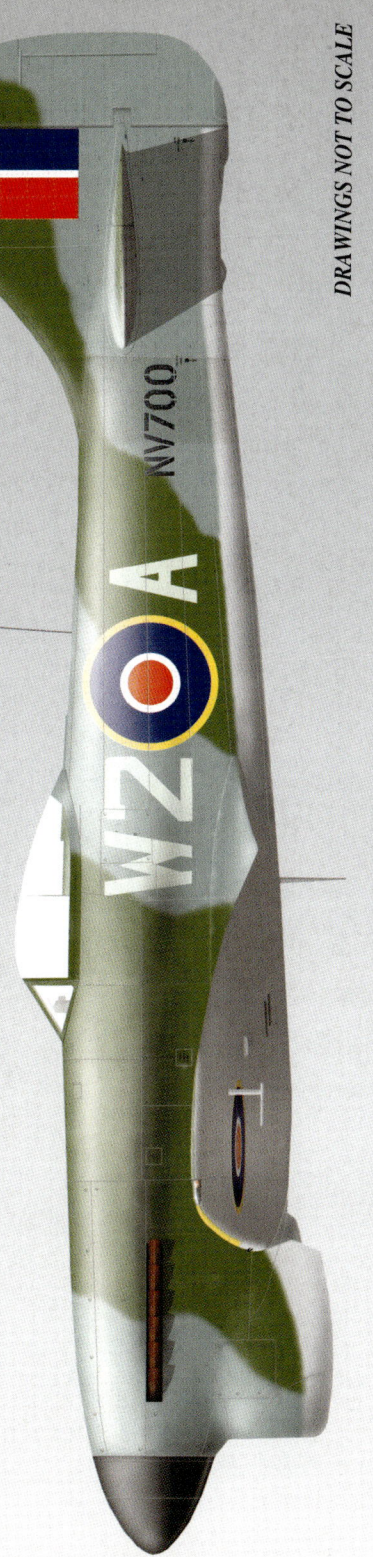

Tempest Mk V NV700 W2-A, 80 Sqn, 2nd TAF. Standard RAF/2nd TAF camouflage – black spinner, fuselage band painted over. While flying this plane S/L Mackie took part in combat on March 2nd but without success.

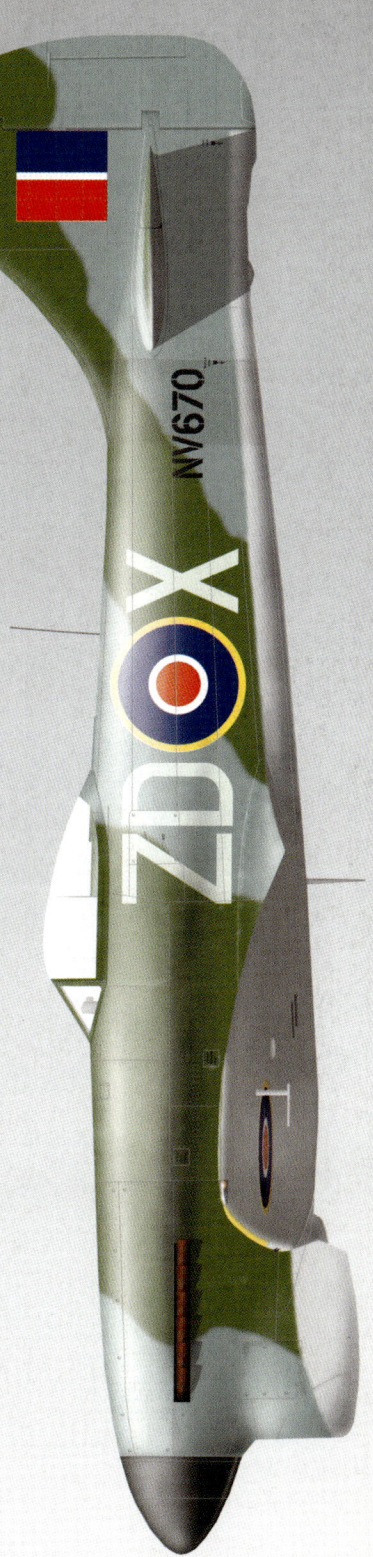

Tempest Mk. V NV670 ZD-X, 222 Sqn, 2nd TAF. Standard RAF/2nd TAF camouflage – black spinner, fuselage band painted over. With this plane F/L McAuliffe shot down a Bf 109 from III/JG 27, although his personal mount was ZD-S NV774.

An Ordinary Day in 1945

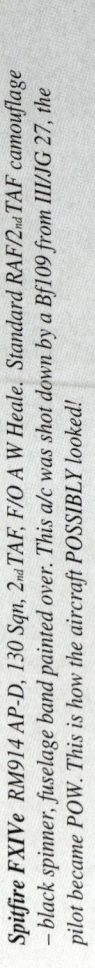

DRAWINGS NOT TO SCALE

Spitfire FXIVe RM914 AP-D, 130 Sqn, 2nd TAF, F/O A W Heale. Standard RAF/2nd TAF camouflage – black spinner, fuselage band painted over. This a/c was shot down by a Bf109 from III/JG 27, the pilot became POW. This is how the aircraft POSSIBLY looked!

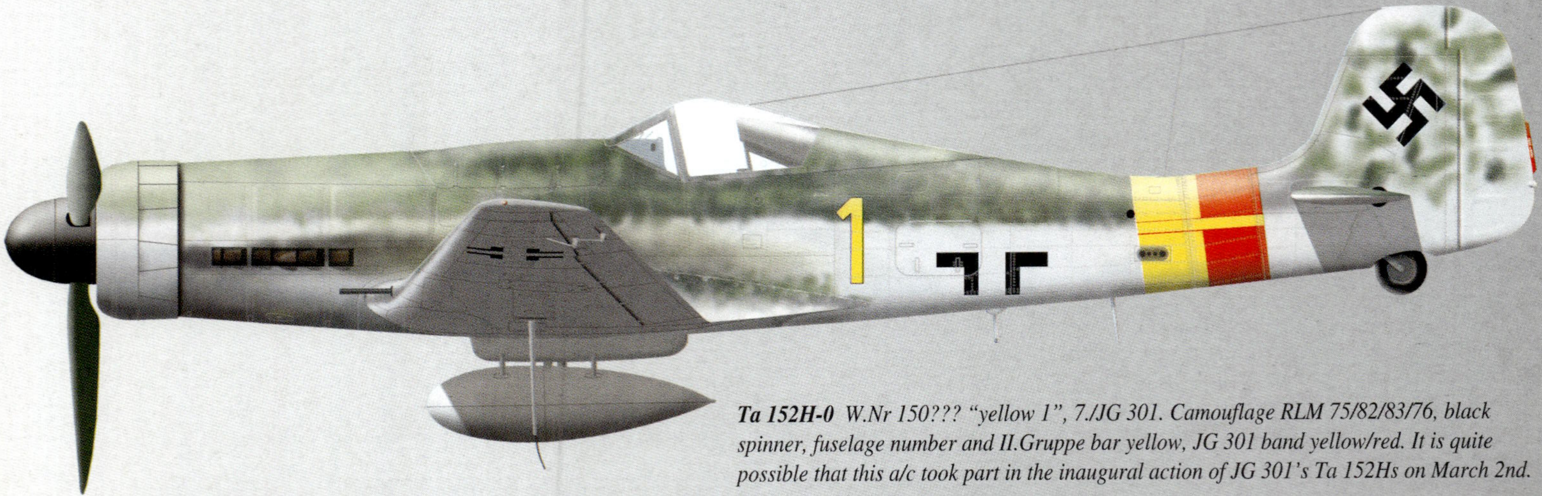

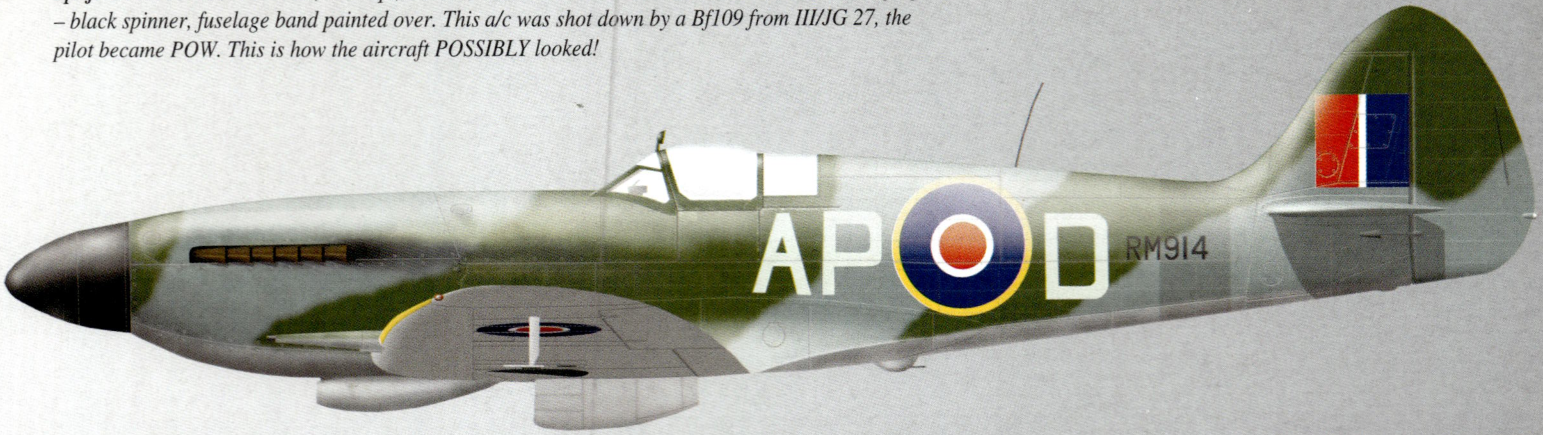

Ta 152H-0 W.Nr 150??? "yellow 1", 7./JG 301. Camouflage RLM 75/82/83/76, black spinner, fuselage number and II.Gruppe bar yellow, JG 301 band yellow/red. It is quite possible that this a/c took part in the inaugural action of JG 301's Ta 152Hs on March 2nd.

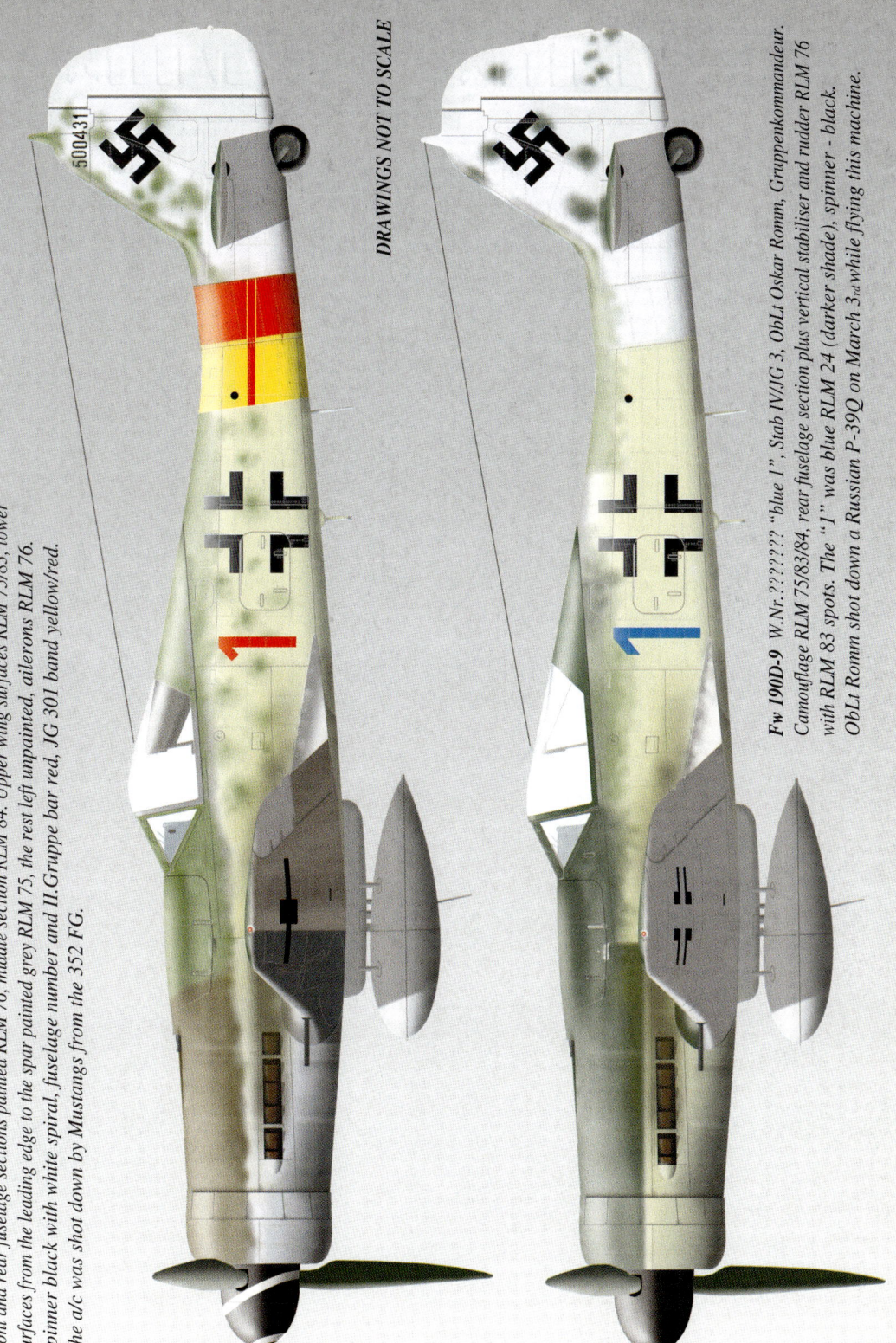

DRAWINGS NOT TO SCALE

Fw 190D-9 W.Nr.500431 "red 1", 6./JG 301, Ln Walter Kropp, Staffelkapitän. Upper fuselage RLM 81/82, front and rear fuselage sections painted RLM 76, middle section RLM 84. Upper wing surfaces RLM 75/83, lower surfaces from the leading edge to the spar painted grey RLM 75, the rest left unpainted, ailerons RLM 76. Spinner black with white spiral, fuselage number and II.Gruppe red, JG 301 band yellow/red. The a/c was shot down by Mustangs from the 352 FG.

Fw 190D-9 W.Nr. ?????? "blue 1", Stab IV/JG 3, ObLt Oskar Romm, Gruppenkommandeur. Camouflage RLM 75/83/84, rear fuselage section plus vertical stabiliser and rudder RLM 76 with RLM 83 spots. The "1" was blue RLM 24 (darker shade), spinner - black. ObLt Romm shot down a Russian P-39Q on March 3rd while flying this machine.

An Ordinary Day in 1945

An Ordinary Day in 1945
DRAWINGS NOT TO SCALE

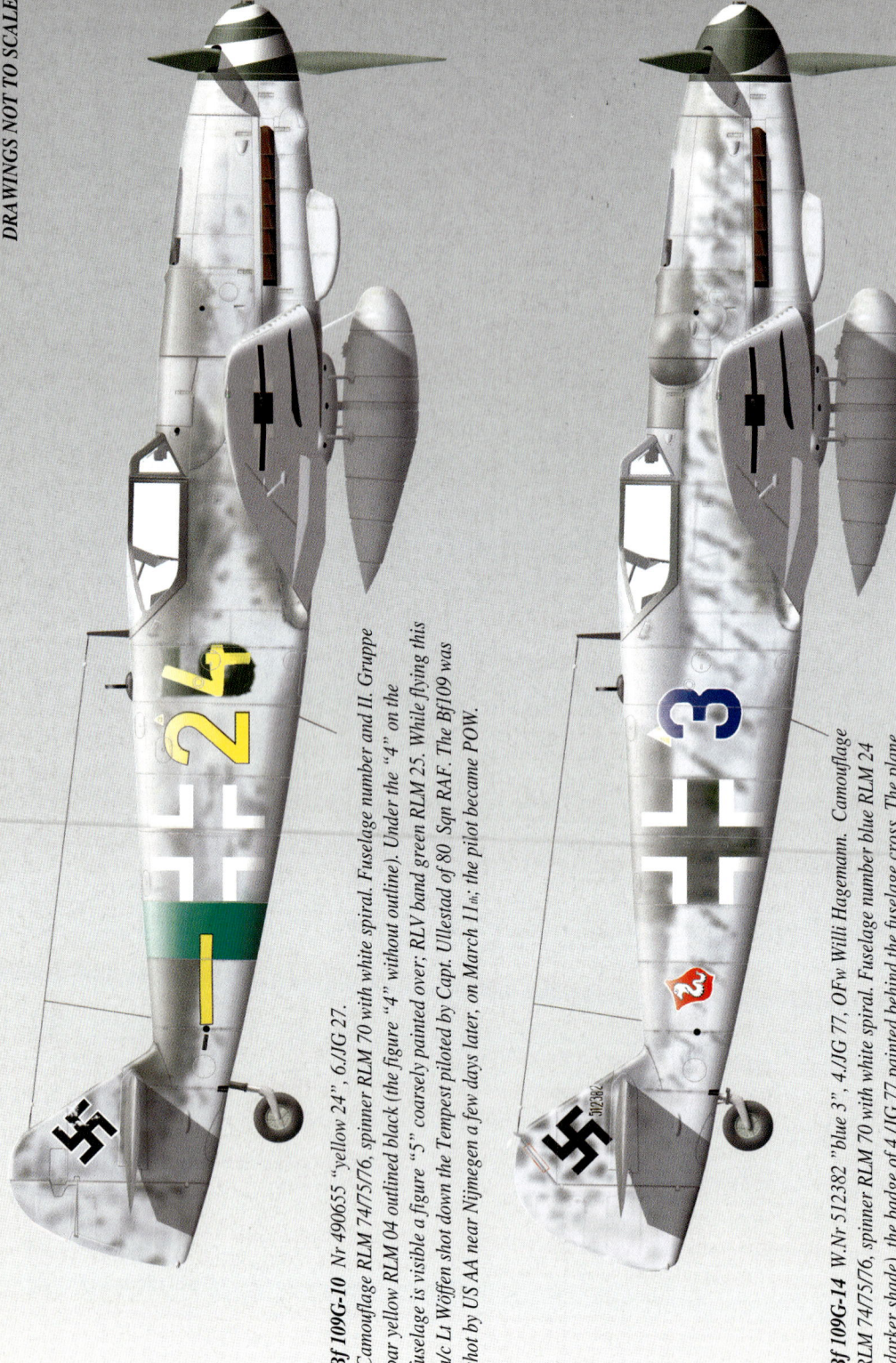

Bf 109G-10 Nr 490655 "yellow 24", 6./JG 27. Camouflage RLM 74/75/76, spinner RLM 70 with white spiral. Fuselage number and II. Gruppe bar yellow RLM 04 outlined black (the figure "4" without outline). Under the "4" on the fuselage is visible a figure "5" coarsely painted over; RLV band green RLM 25. While flying this a/c Lt Wöffen shot down the Tempest piloted by Capt. Ullestad of 80 Sqn RAF. The Bf109 was shot by US AA near Nijmegen a few days later, on March 11th; the pilot became POW.

Bf 109G-14 W.Nr 512382 "blue 3", 4./JG 77, OFw Willi Hagemann. Camouflage RLM 74/75/76, spinner RLM 70 with white spiral. Fuselage number blue RLM 24 (darker shade), the badge of 4./JG 77 painted behind the fuselage cross. The plane was damaged by 45% in a crash landing at Prerau, the pilot was wounded.

DRAWINGS NOT TO SCALE

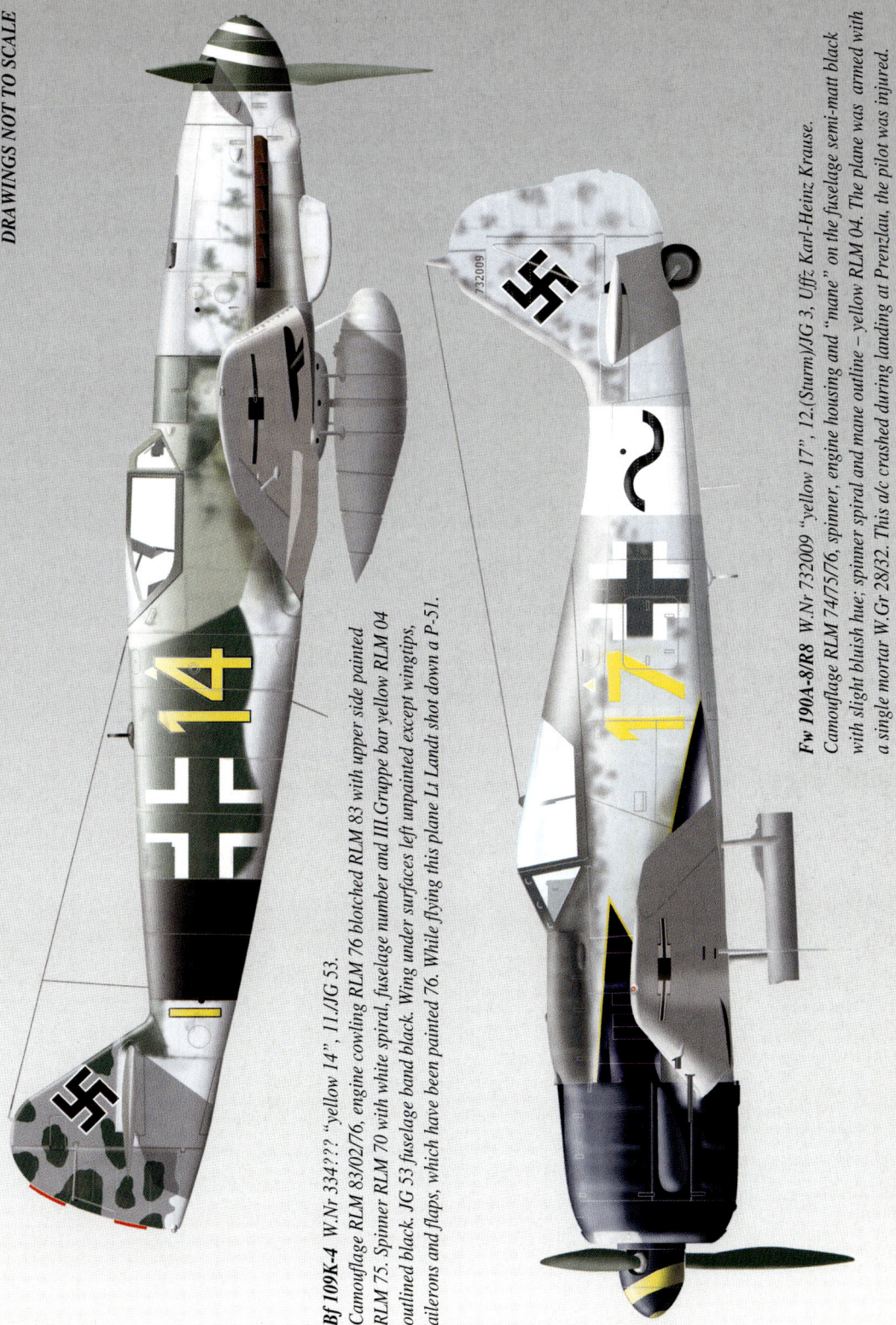

Bf 109K-4 W.Nr 334??? "yellow 14", 11./JG 53. Camouflage RLM 83/02/76, engine cowling RLM 76 blotched RLM 83 with upper side painted RLM 75. Spinner RLM 70 with white spiral, fuselage number and III.Gruppe bar yellow RLM 04 outlined black. JG 53 fuselage band black. Wing under surfaces left unpainted except wingtips, ailerons and flaps, which have been painted 76. While flying this plane Lt Landt shot down a P-51.

Fw 190A-8/R8 W.Nr 732009 "yellow 17", 12.(Sturm)/JG 3, Uffz Karl-Heinz Krause. Camouflage RLM 74/75/76, spinner, engine housing and "mane" on the fuselage semi-matt black with slight bluish hue; spinner spiral and mane outline – yellow RLM 04. The plane was armed with a single mortar W.Gr 28/32. This a/c crashed during landing at Prenzlau, the pilot was injured.

An Ordinary Day in 1945

An Ordinary Day in 1945

DRAWINGS NOT TO SCALE

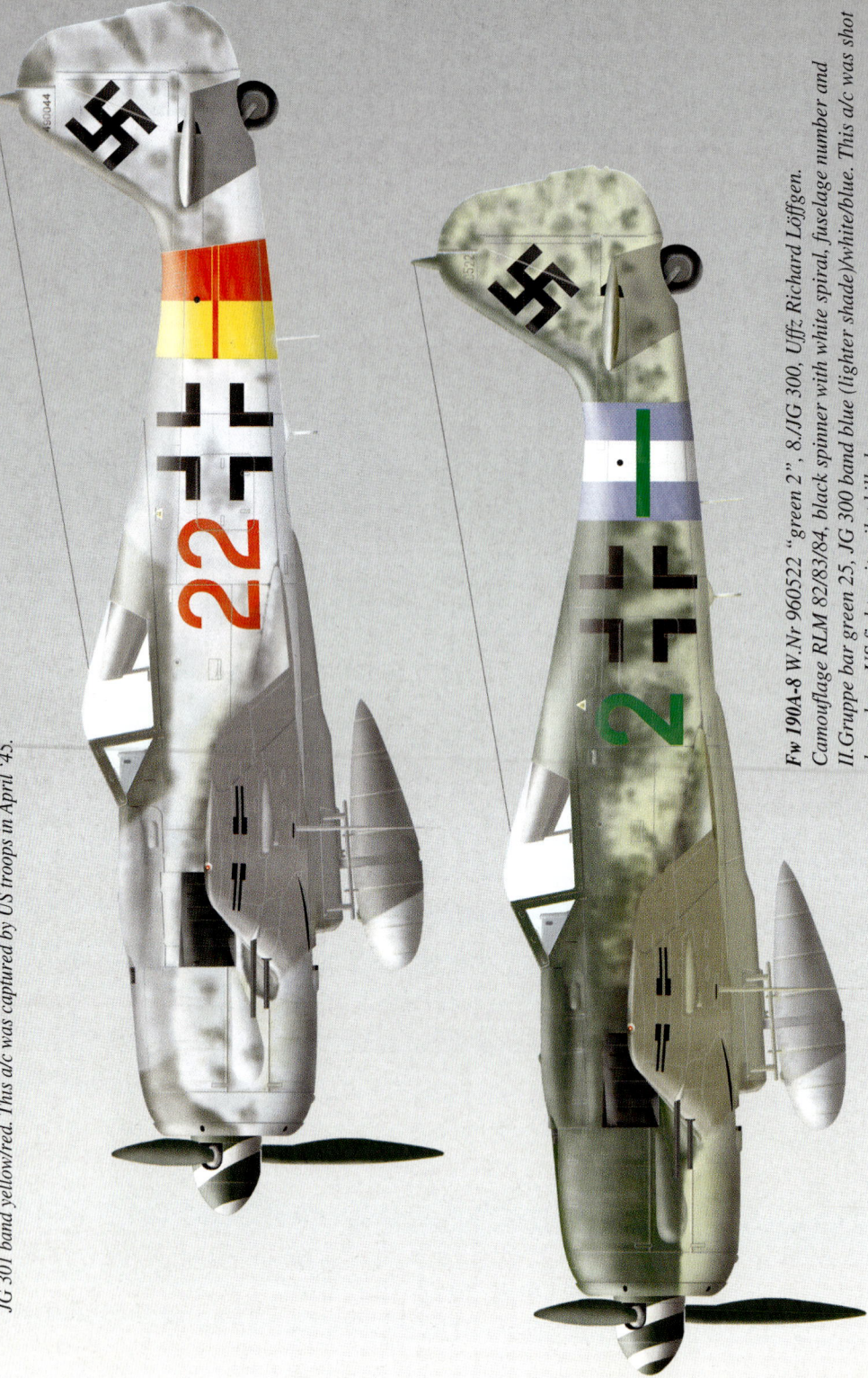

Fw 190A-9 W.Nr 490044 "red 22", 6./JG 301, pilot unknown. Camouflage RLM 74/75/76, black spinner with white spiral, fuselage number and II.Gruppe bar red, JG 301 band yellow/red. This a/c was captured by US troops in April '45.

Fw 190A-8 W.Nr 960522 "green 2", 8./JG 300, Uffz Richard Löffgen. Camouflage RLM 82/83/84, black spinner with white spiral, fuselage number and II.Gruppe bar green 25, JG 300 band blue (lighter shade)/white/blue. This a/c was shot down by a US fighter, its pilot killed.

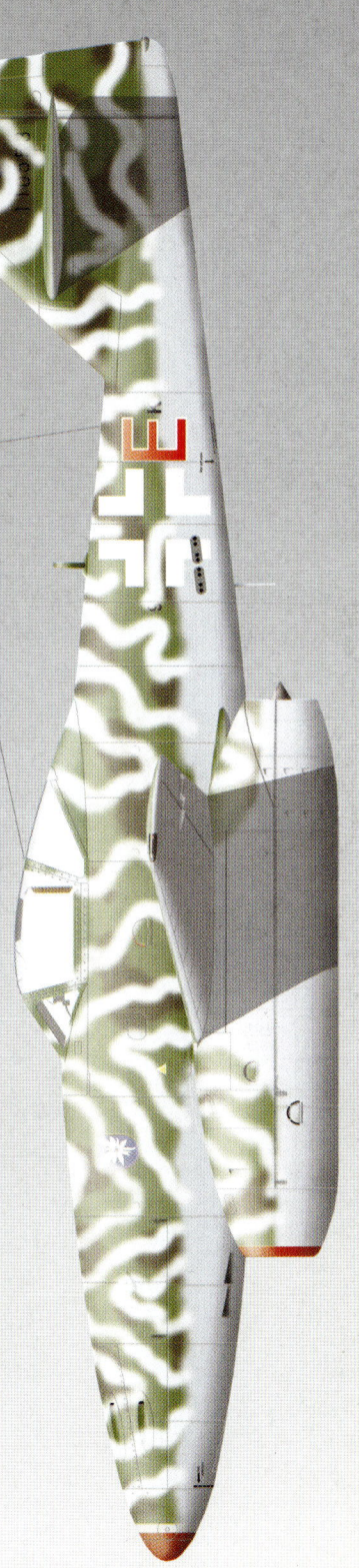

An Ordinary Day in 1945

Me 262A-2a W.Nr 110913 B3+YL, 3./KG(J) 54, Fhr Heinrich Griems. Camouflage RLM 81/82/76, fuselage nose, individual letter and vertical stabiliser tip painted red. This a/c was shot down by a Mustang from the 354 FG flown by Capt. Peters, its pilot KIA. This how the a/c POSSIBLY looked!

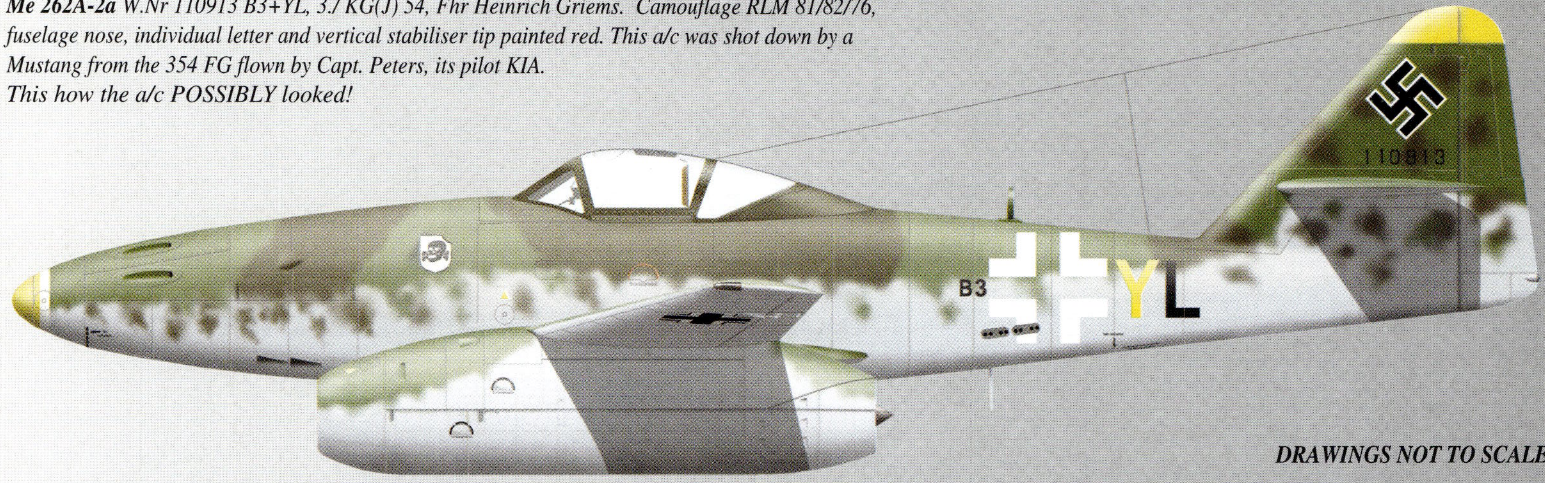

Me 262A-2a W.Nr 110553 9K+EN, 5./KG 51, Hptm. Fritz Abel. Camouflage RLM 81/82/76, with wide wavy RLM 76 stripes on upper and side surfaces. Fuselage nose, front of engine nacelles, individual letter and vertical stabiliser tip painted red. The a/c was shot down by an F-6 from the 107 TRS piloted by 1st/Lt Dunmire, the pilot killed. This how the a/c POSSIBLY looked!

DRAWINGS NOT TO SCALE

An Ordinary Day in 1945

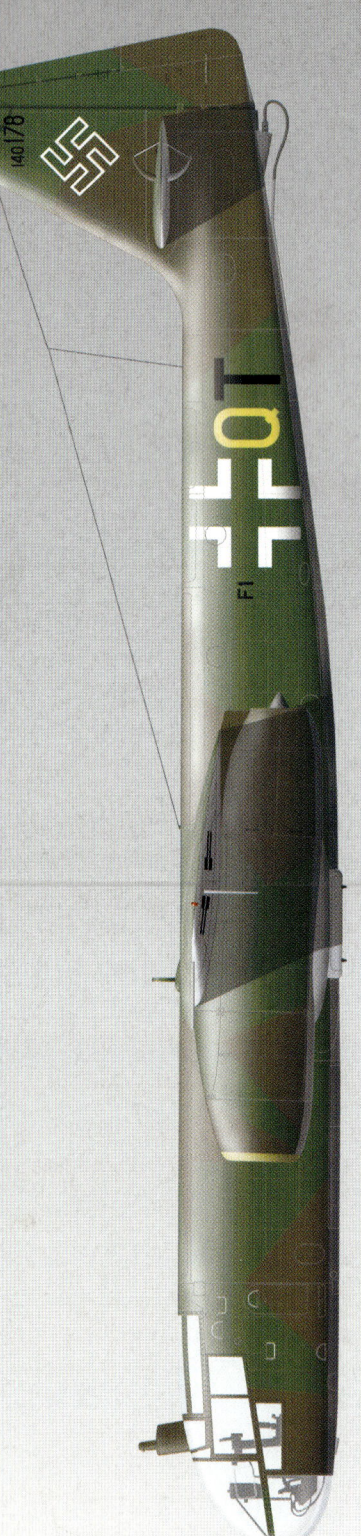

Ar 234B-2 W.Nr. 140178 F1+QT, 9./KG 76, Lt Eberhard Rögele. Camouflage RLM 81/82/76. Front of engine nacelles and individual letters yellow RLM 04. The plane was shot down on March 2nd by F/L G. W. Varley of 222 Sqn RAF. This how the a/c POSSIBLY looked!

DRAWINGS NOT TO SCALE

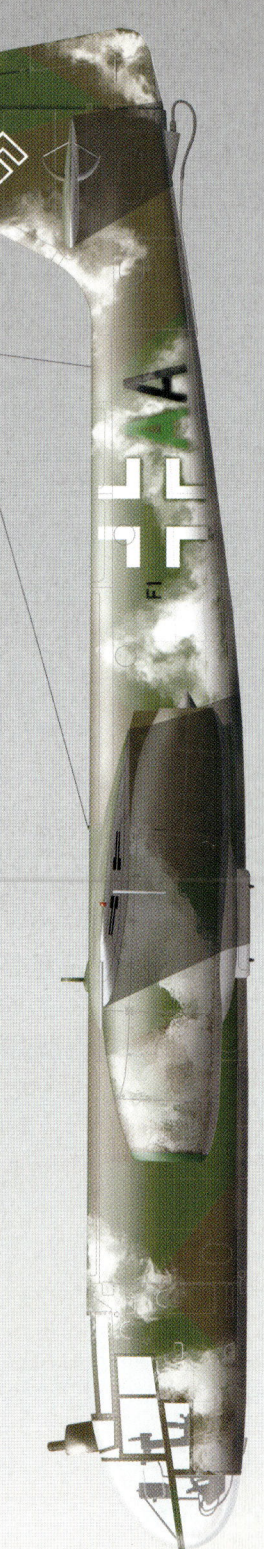

Ar 234B-2 W.Nr. 140113 F1+AA Stab KG 76. Camouflage RLM 81/82/76 partially painted over with whitewash or RLM 76. The individual letter "A" and front edge of engine nacelles painted green RLM 25. In this machine ObLt Kowalewski led the attack against the Remagen bridge on March 17th; it is quite possible that on March 2nd the plane wore the same camouflage. The plane was captured by the RAF and transferred to England, where it was given the serial VH530.